THE HAZARD

FROM DANGEROUS

EXOTIC DISEASES

THE HAZARD FROM DANGEROUS EXOTIC DISEASES

by

John C. N. Westwood, M.B., B.Chir.,
Professor and Chairman,
Department of Microbiology and Immunology,
School of Medicine, Faculty of Health Sciences,
University of Ottawa, Ottawa, Canada.

Softcover reprint of the hardcover 1st edition 1980

First published 1980 by

THE MACMILLAN PRESS LTD
London and Basingstoke

Associated Companies throughout the world

ISBN 978-1-349-05279-0   ISBN 978-1-349-05277-6 (eBook)
DOI 10.1007/978-1-349-05277-6

Published in the United States and its dependencies by The Franklin Institute Press, Philadelphia, Pa.

Filmset by Vantage Photosetting Co. Ltd., Southampton and London

Contents

List of Illustrations

List of Tables

Acknowledgements

This book is based upon an extensive study of the relevant literature interpreted in light of my personal experience as a public health and research virologist, with a major involvement in smallpox research, as well as consultations with present authorities in the problems of control of communicable diseases in North America and Europe.

Particular attention has been paid to the 'new' haemorrhagic virus diseases including Lassa and Ebola-Marburg fevers and most of the established authorities on the control, containment and clinical management of these diseases in Britain and the US have been consulted.

The study was funded by the Ministry of Health of Ontario and I wish to express my sincere appreciation of the financial support received.

I also wish to thank the following authorities for their help and patience under persistent questioning:

Dr E. T. W. Bowen, Special Pathogens Division, Medical Research Establishment, Porton, England

Dr Philip S. Brachman, Director, Bureau of Epidemiology, Center for Disease Control, Atlanta, Georgia, US

Dr Paul Brès, Director, Virus Diseases, WHO, Geneva, Switzerland

Dr A. J. Clayton, Director General, Laboratory Centre for Disease Control, Health and Welfare, Canada

Dr J. L. Conrad, Director, Field Services Division, Center for Disease Control, Atlanta, Georgia, US

Dr H. M. Darlow, Safety Officer (Ret'd.), Medical Research Establishment, Porton, England

Dr R. E. Dixon, Chief, Hospital Infections Branch, Bacterial Diseases Division, Bureau of Epidemiology, Center for Disease Control, Atlanta, Georgia, US

Dr R. T. D. Emond, Consultant in Infectious Diseases, Royal Free and Northern Hospitals, London, and Coppett's Wood Hospital, London, England

Dr R. J. Fallon, Consultant in Laboratory Medicine, Ruchill Hospital, Glasgow, Scotland

Dr Stanley Foster, Center for Disease Control, Atlanta, Georgia, US

Dr N. S. Galbraith, Director, Communicable Disease Surveillance Centre, Public Health Laboratory Service, London, England

Prof H. M. J. Gilles, Professor of Tropical Medicine, Liverpool University, Liverpool, England

Dr Karl Johnson, Chief, Special Pathogens Branch, Center for Disease Control, Atlanta, Georgia, US

Prof H. P. Lambert, Professor of Microbial Diseases, University of London and Consultant Physician, St George's Hospital, London, England

Medical Directory Officer, 59 Kingston Road, South Wimbledon, London, England

Dr H. E. Parry, Consultant Physician, Infectious Diseases, Fazakerley Hospital, Liverpool, England

Prof S. R. Pattyn, Prince Leopold Institute for Tropical Diseases, Antwerp, Belgium

Dr A. W. Pearson, Director, Public Health Laboratory, Portsmouth, England

Dr I. W. Pinkerton, Consultant Physician, Department of Infectious Diseases, Ruchill Hospital, Glasgow, Scotland

Dr J. B. Selkon, Director, Public Health Laboratory, Newcastle-upon-Tyne, England

Dr D. I. H. Simpson, Director, Special Pathogens Division, Medical Research Establishment, Porton, England

Dr C. E. Gordon Smith, Dean, London School of Hygiene and Tropical Medicine and Chairman of Board, Public Health Laboratory Service, England

Dr R. A. Sprenger, Senior Consultant, Quarantine and Regulatory, Medical Services Branch, Health and Welfare, Canada

Dr G. van der Groen, Prince Leopold Institute for Tropical Diseases, Antwerp, Belgium

Dr R. V. Walley, Consultant Physician, Communicable Diseases, Ham Green Hospital, Bristol, England

Sir Robert Williams, Director, Public Health Laboratory Service, London, England

Dr Susan Young, Communicable Disease Surveillance Centre, Public Health Laboratory Service, London, England

I also wish to express particular thanks to: Dr D. I. H. Simpson, Director, Special Pathogens Division, M.R.E. Porton, who led to WHO team investigating the Sudan epidemic of Ebola fever, for his constant help throughout the year and for reading the original report before its submission to the Ontario Ministry of Health. Dr E. T. W. Bowen of the Special Pathogens Division, M.R.E. Porton, for his help and advice on the virological aspects of Lassa and Ebola-Marburg disease; for permission to use his published and unpublished data and the full text of his Ph.D. thesis and, finally, for reading the original report before its submission to the Ontario Ministry of Health.

Extensive discussions with these two workers and with Dr Karl Johnson of CDC, Atlanta, were of inestimable value in amplifying their official WHO reports with impressions and factual data obtained in Sudan and Zaire respectively.

My sincere thanks to Dr Robert Harris, Director, MRE, Porton, for permission to use the library and facilities of the Establishment as headquarters for this work, and to Dr David Crichton, Air Commodore, R.A.F. (Ret'd.), for reading and criticizing the draft report.

Thanks should also go to Vickers Medical Company, Basingstoke, Hampshire and Martindale Protection Ltd, London, for supplying photographs of their equipment. Figures 1–4 are courtesy of the World Health Organization in Geneva.

Finally, I have made free use of ideas discussed at the meetings of the Canadian Federal Working Party on the Coordinated Response to National Communicable Disease Emergencies, and particularly those of Dr A. J. Clayton and Dr R. Sprenger. Dr Sprenger's lucid written submissions to the working party have proved a most valuable source of ideas and information.

Section One

Background Situation

1

Cause for Alarm

When Marburg virus suddenly struck 'out of the blue' in 1967 in three European cities not only was the episode frightening to a generation long considered safe from dangerous epidemic diseases but it profoundly shocked the medical profession. The haemorrhagic syndrome, the lethality and the transmissibility to staff attending the patients were unprecedented and virologists were startled to discover that the *aetiological* agent was a previously unknown virus of bizarre morphology and unique antigenic constitution.

The immediate source of the outbreak was quickly identified as one particular batch of vervet monkeys from Uganda, imported for producing tissue cultures for vaccines, but intensive research during the next few years failed to uncover the original reservoir where the monkeys themselves derived their infection. Even the reappearance of the virus eight years later, which resulted in the death of a student in South Africa, failed to reveal its origins.

This virus, appearing at a time when major fatal epidemics had been virtually eliminated from the developed countries of the West, served as a sharp reminder that all was not known in the realm of virology. The subsequent dramatic appearance of Lassa fever in 1969 and its spread to scientific investigators in the US hammered home the message and the lethal outbreak of Ebola fever in Zaire and Sudan in 1976 set the final seal upon it.

While these events were serious, their implications in respect of susceptible populations in the world outside Africa were even more so. In all three cases, the initial events indicated an exceptional communicability and, in the case of Lassa and Ebola fevers, a high lethality to health care personnel infected as a result of caring for sick patients.

During the few weeks of its epidemic course, Ebola fever had spread from its remote epicentres in Central Africa to cause deaths in Kinshasa in southwest Zaire and in Khartoum in northern Sudan – a span of 3,000 km – while Lassa fever had been introduced on several occasions into Europe and the US. It was clear that with the growing volume of freight and passenger air-transportation, the introduction of these diseases to countries outside Africa would be increasing, and they could release the viruses into crowded urbanized populations totally unprotected by either individual or herd immunity to infection.

The episodes which occurred in the 10 years since the first appearance of Marburg virus disease had not led to extensive community epidemics outside the African endemo-epidemic areas but the ready infection of staff caring for patients and the high lethality of the diseases posed a formidable public health threat. The possibility of an uncontrollable pandemic in the pattern of influenza, but with a case-fatality rate of between 30 and 80 per cent, could not be ruled out on the available information. Many governments were faced with the need to develop contingency plans and to consider building high-security isolation facilities for the management of cases or suspects.

The possibilities for disaster were obvious but data were lacking for a reliable estimate of the immediacy of the threat and the early response in all countries affected was improvisation to deal with actual or suspected introductions. Under these circumstances, and in the full glare of media coverage, decisions regarding appropriate level of response are determined as much by emotional and political considerations as by scientific analysis of the threat. Even after the immediate incident has passed, the influence of the emotional and political factors remains since these will flare up again at each subsequent crisis. Only the deadening effect of repetition and habituation will counter this effect.

Apart from these considerations a reliable scientific working estimate of the threat is critically important. Under-reaction could be extremely dangerous both to the community and to the health-care staff who must transport, investigate, nurse and treat cases, while over-reaction may be self-defeating.

Dangerous, highly communicable diseases require efficient public health procedures for their control and containment and these must be backed by adquate isolation facilities. If, however, these facilities are over-elaborate in design, their cost can become so formidable that they are never built. In Canada, the danger was first recognized in 1972 when the Canadian Armed Forces were asked to repatriate a suspected case from Nigeria and a similar request occurred in 1974. With the prospect of the 1976 Olympic Games to be held in Montreal, a federal working party was appointed to formulate functional plans for an isolation facility in association with the National Defence Medical Centre in Ottawa. After two years, the plans were never fulfilled because of cost. In 1976, an Ontario Government working party carried out a similar function without results, and in 1977, the federal government announced its intention of proceeding with its originally planned facility. Again the project was dropped because of the expense. In 1979, the issue was again being discussed at the Provincial level.

After seven years of awareness, there is still no satisfactory isolation facility in the entire country to back the Canadian Contingency Plan prepared in 1977. In the UK, where structural planning was on a lower key and where disused wings of old, underutilized fever hospitals could be suitably modified, progress has been faster. Six designated facilities have been completed. In continental Europe, the only purpose-designed, high-security facility built to counter the threat of smallpox is at the Robert Koch Institute in West Berlin. In the US, a single facility exists at the old biological warfare establishment at Fort Detrick with a minor two-bed isolation unit for smallpox cases at the Staten Island Hospital for merchant seamen.

Awareness of the danger is not enough to stimulate governments to spend the money needed to meet the threat. Only repetition will achieve that result and it is no coincidence that the UK, with its repeated exposure to suspected cases, is ahead of every other nation in its response.

The pressure on other countries will, however, grow. Three 'new' lethal diseases have already been released in Africa while two newly encountered haemorrhagic fevers are spreading through populous regions of South America. Even the old enemy yellow fever has been given a fresh stimulus to epidemic expression in West Africa and in regions of South America.

More 'new' diseases will certainly be encountered in the

future and air transportation has ensured that no corner of the world can be considered so remote that it cannot be reached by an infected individual during the incubation period of any of these diseases. The hazard is clearly greatest in the highly urbanized, developed communities because of the density and mobility of their populations, and because the use of their technology and expertise in the remote area developments ensures continued and increasingly frequent travel to and from these areas.

Since the dangers will increase with each passing year, it would seem highly desirable to make a thorough scientific assessment of the present and future hazard from exotic diseases so that a rational response may be developed at a practical cost and adequate protection be established.

The following facts may help to establish the wisdom of this course of action.

During the Asian influenza pandemic of 1957–58, it was estimated that some 70 million of the 180 million population of the US contracted the disease over an eight-week period – an attack rate of 39 per cent. The peak incidence was about 12 million cases a week and it was estimated that about 5 million people were confined to bed with the disease at any one time. The case fatality rate of 'Asian influenza' was trivial yet over 60,000 deaths were attributed to it in the US.

The 1918–19 'Spanish' influenza pandemic is now legendary and the generally accepted estimate of its death-toll is 15–20 million across the world – almost 1 per cent of the total world population at that time. Yet in that pandemic, the case-fatality rate averaged only 3 per cent. The consequences of pandemic spread of an equally transmissible disease with the 88 per cent lethality of the Zaire strain of Ebola virus, or even the 25 per cent lethality of Lassa virus, would be truly formidable not only by the direct death rate but also through the inevitable break-down of world services including power and food distribution.

Could such an event occur? The answer is undoubtedly 'yes'. What is the likelihood of its occurring? The immediate answer lies in the present nature of the newly emergent diseases and is the purpose of the detailed analysis in Section Two. Decisions regarding the appropriate level of response in immediate public health contingency planning, and in the development of isolation facilities and diagnostic and patient management procedures depend on the likelihood of the newly emergent diseases becoming pandemic.

The study reported in this monograph was funded by the Ontario Ministry of Health and was designed to provide a scientific basis for rational response. No attempt has been made to analyse the emotional, social and political factors which also bear upon that response nor has the report been extended beyond an assessment of the present threat in the light of the known behaviour of the exotic diseases. It will become evident, however, that the situation is far from static and the long-term possibilities may be very different from those of the immediate future. These will be considered in a subsequent publication.

2

Assessment of the Threat

In terms of threat to Western communities, the events of the past few years have focused attention on Marburg, Lassa and Ebola fevers in their capacity as new, lethal and highly communicable diseases, but they are not the only diseases which merit consideration. Other diseases such as Legionnaires' disease and Rift Valley fever are both newly emergent and dangerous while some of the older diseases such as smallpox and plague cannot be ignored. Preliminary scrutiny suggests that the diseases listed in Table I should be examined in terms both of their epidemic threat to human communities and their ecological threat. The ecological threat is posed by the possibility of establishing the diseases in previously uninfected potential reservoirs in regional fauna outside their present geographical limits.

The primary concern is undoubtedly the epidemic threat and it is necessary to understand its nature and the basic epidemiological factors which may enhance or limit it.

Epidemic potential

In its simplest form, transmission of infectious disease requires a source or reservoir, a susceptible host and a mechanism of transmission. In human disease the susceptible host is human, but the source may be inanimate, as in the saprozoonoses typified by histoplasmosis, or may be an animal species as in the zoonoses. Transmission may occur by physical contact of which the closest and most direct is sexual, including kissing and caressing, or by the agency of an intermediate vehicle which may be a person, an arthropod vector or inanimate. This type of transmission is indirect and does not entail physical ccontact between reservoir and susceptible new host.

TABLE 1   Epidemic threat

Viral Haemorrhagic Fevers

Transmission category	
Airborne and contact	Smallpox
Mosquito-borne	Yellow fever Haemorrhagic dengue Chikungunya fever Rift Valley fever
Tick-borne	Crimean-Congo Kyasanur Omsk haemorrhagic fever Korean haemorrhagic fever with renal syndrome
Rodent-associated	Argentinian haemorrhagic fever Bolivian haemorrhagic fever Lassa fever
Unknown	Marburg fever Ebola fever
Other diseases	
	Herpes B Plague Cholera Legionnaires' disease

Persons as vehicles

When a person acts as a vehicle the mechanism may be a purely mechanical transfer on contaminated fingers or may involve actual colonization of the intermediary who thus becomes a *carrier* in the technical sense, and may constitute a reservoir in continuing the infection chain.

Inanimate vehicles

Inanimate vehicles of infection may be grouped under food, water, air and fomites; when considering epidemic threat in developed communities, the air is undoubtedly the most important of these. Although food-borne disease is by no means fully controlled even under the best conditions, for example, the frequency of individual outbreaks of food-poisoning and the general increase in salmonellosis in recent years, major uncontrollable epidemics of food-borne disease should not occur in developed communities subject to modern hygienic standards. Similarly, major epidemics should not occur from agents spread by the water-borne route, although limited outbreaks of such diseases as Hepatitis A will certainly be encountered.

Airborne infection, however, is in a different category and its uncontrollability is obvious in the behaviour of influenza on any scale from the endemic to the pandemic. There can be no doubt that transmissibility by the respiratory route is by far the most important single factor to be considered when assessing the epidemic potential of the diseases under consideration.

Arthropod vectors

Arthropod vectors of disease occur as intermediate hosts in a wide range of zoonotic diseases in which man may become involved, usually as an incidental host who is not part of the primary infection chain. This is the case with most of the mosquito-borne viral encephalitides of Africa and North America and the tick-borne haemorrhagic fevers of Eastern Europe and Asia. Although this incidental involvement usually gives rise to sporadic cases rather than extensive epidemics, large numbers of human cases may sometimes occur even in the absence of person-to-person spread. This was probably the case in the extensive Nigerian yellow fever outbreak of 1969–70 mediated by *Aedes simpsoni* where some 100,000 cases were estimated to have occurred.

The greatest epidemic threat to man occurs when man himself becomes the reservoir in a specifically human infection chain independent of the zoonotic animal reservoir. The classical example is the devastating urban yellow fever of the seventeenth, eighteenth and nineteenth centuries which was transmitted by peri-domestic *Aedes aegypti* mosquitos through the human population independently of the sylvatic monkey reservoirs maintained by the high-flying forest canopy mosquitos.

Even where an arthropod vector forms an essential link in the infection chain, epidemic spread, although it may be devastating, is geographically limited by the distribution of the vector. In yellow fever this confines the disease to tropical and subtropical zones. This limitation is broken only when the vector-borne mechanism of transmission is also short-circuited by the development of direct person-to-person transmission. Such an occurrence is seen in the epidemics of pneumonic plague where the bubonic rat-flea-rat and rat-flea-man transmission cycles become supplanted by direct person-to-person respiratory transmission of the pneumonic form of the disease. Such a transformation of the transmission mechanism releases the disease from constraints set by the geographical distribution of animal reservoir and vector alike and is the real danger to be feared from the threatening newly-emergent diseases which are without exception zoonoses with identified or presumed animal reservoirs.

It seems clear that the most critical factor which governs the epidemic threat from any of these diseases is its ability to spread directly from person-to-person by the respiratory route. The magnitude of this threat may be gauged by the behaviour of measles when introduced into a fully susceptible population. In 1951, a seaman incubating measles introduced the disease into southern Greenland and in the ensuing epidemic no fewer than 4,257 persons out of a total population of 4,262 contracted the disease.

Ecological threat

Although epidemic potential must clearly dominate the present assessment of threat, the ecological possibilities cannot be ignored. In 1900, plague was introduced into California, probably by plague-infected rats going ashore from ships in San Francisco harbour. During the ensuing years, infection spread beyond the confines of the city and entered the indigenous rodent population. Since that time, it has spread relentlessly east to the extent that the western US is now one of the three major endemic plague foci in the world. The incidence of human plague in the US is extremely low – fewer than 20 cases per year – but its presence nevertheless constitutes a continuous threat to the population with the disturbing possibility of epidemic pneumonic plague always in the background and the virtual certainty that infection will ultimately reach the rat populations of the densely urbanized Eastern seaboard. Certain major viral haemorrhagic fevers are maintained in rodent reservoirs and there is, as yet, no information regarding the susceptibility of the enormous range of rodent species indigenous to regions beyond their endemic areas. Although data are lacking for any reasonable assessment of the risk involved, the possible danger should not be ignored in planning appropriate public health response.

3

Candidate Diseases

Viral haemorrhagic fevers

While haemorrhages associated with severe infectious disease
are not uncommon – for instance, in haemorrhagic varicella or
the Waterhouse-Friderichsen syndrome in acute meningococ-
caemia – the occurrence of haemorrhagic tendency as a characteristic clinical feature has led to the grouping together of
certain viral diseases under the heading of Viral Haemorrhagic
Fevers (VHF).

As shown in Table 2, they are a heterogeneous group of
diverse aetiology and wide, but often strictly regional, distribution. All but smallpox are zoonoses or are presumed so and most
are arthropod transmitted. Only smallpox, yellow fever and
dengue were recognized as human infections before 1930 and
the haemorrhagic syndrome in dengue did not appear in
epidemic form until 1953. Despite the tens of thousands of
people who have been killed by these diseases during the last 30
years, none have engendered a degree of alarm in developed
communities in any way comparable to that which followed the
emergence of Lassa and Ebola fevers.

Smallpox

Smallpox is one of the most ancient epidemic diseases of man
and up to a century ago was of worldwide distribution.

Although the classical clinical picture is that of a highly toxic
exanthem with an abundant centrifugal rash affecting mainly
the head, face and extremities of the limbs, the disease is a true
haemorrhagic fever, with skin haemorrhages varying from
petechiae to widespread haemorrhagic necrosis and frank

TABLE 2 Viral haemorrhagic fevers

Transmission category	Disease	Year recognized	Virus group	Arthropod vector(s)	Mammalian reservoir	Geographic distribution
Airborne and contact	Smallpox	(prehistory)	Poxvirus	None	Man	Eradicated
Mosquito-borne	Yellow fever	1647	Flavivirus	*Sylvan neotropical Haemagogus spp. Sabethes*	Monkeys Cebus spp. Ateles spp. Alouatta spp.	Tropical Central and S. America
				Sylvan african Aedes africanus Aedes simpsoni	Sercopithecus spp. Colubus	Tropical Africa
				Urban *Aedes aegypti*	Man	Tropical Central and S. America and Africa
	Haemorrhagic dengue	1953	Flavivirus	Rural: *Aedes albopictus*	Sylvan primates (not proved)	Entire tropics
				Urban: *Aedes aegypti*	Man	
	Chikungunya fever	1952	Flavivirus	*Aedes africanus Aedes aegypti*	? Monkeys	India and S.E. Asia Africa
	Rift Valley fever	1930	Flavivirus	*Aedes caballus Culex fatigans Culex theileri* etc.	? Rodents Secondary-domestic sheep and cattle	Egypt, Sudan, E. and S. Africa

	Disease	Year	Virus	Vector	Host	Location
Tick-borne or Mite-borne	Crimean-Congo Haemorrhagic fever Hazara fever	1944	Flavivirus	*Hyalomma marginatus* *H. onatoliem*	Small mammals ?Cattle	USSR, Bulgaria Pakistan, Africa
	Kyasanur Forest disease	1957	Flavivirus	*Haemaphysalis spp.* *Ixodes spp.*	Small mammals Langur and Macacus monkeys	India especially Mysore
	Omsk H.F.	1945	Flavivirus	*Dermacentor pictus* *Dermacentor spp.*	Muskrats	Siberia
	Korean H.F. = H.F. with Renal syndrome	1930–1951	Unknown	Unknown	Field mice and voles (*Apodemus* spp.)	Eastern USSR Korea, Japan, Czechoslovakia, Yugoslavia
Rodent-associated	Argentinian H.F.	1943	Arenavirus	None	*Calomys* spp.	Argentina
	Bolivian H.F.	1959	Arenavirus	None	*Calomys callosus*	Bolivia
	Lassa fever	1969	Arenavirus	None	Multimammate rat (*Mastomys natalensis*)	N.W. Africa ?E. Africa
Unknown	Marburg fever	1967	Marburg	?	? Monkeys susceptible	Africa ?Regions
	Ebola fever	1976	Marburg	?	? Bats suspect	S. Sudan N.E. Zaire

bleeding from body orifices in the malignant form of the disease.

Smallpox is the only viral haemorrhagic fever which is an exclusively human disease. Man constitutes the reservoir and the mode of transmission is via the respiratory route from person-to-person without the intervention of any vector. The virus is exceptionally hardy and is particularly resistant to drying so that in the airborne state and in dust it may remain fully infectious for long periods.

Although the disease has now been declared to be eradicated (the last known case recovered by 7 October 1977 and the agreed two-year waiting period was successfully completed on 7 October 1979 without another known case) it still merits detailed consideration in Section Two.

Yellow fever

Yellow fever, the prototype of the vector-borne haemorrhagic fevers gives its name to the genus 'Flavivirus' of the Group B Arboviruses. The disease exists in two forms: the urban form, which was originally recognized and elucidated by the US Yellow Fever Commission of 1900, and the sylvan form whose existence was discovered during the 1930s after urban yellow fever had been controlled.

It is now clear that the sylvan form of the disease reflects the true reservoir for the virus which is maintained in the monkey population of the jungle canopies and transmitted by species of mosquitos inhabiting the treetops. These mosquitos do not usually bite man but may do so in particular circumstances. Most of the resulting human infections remain as isolated incidents but, if the victim should introduce the virus into an urban community which is infested with the peridomestic *Aedes aegypti* mosquito, the classical man-mosquito-man cycle of urban yellow fever may be initiated and will run its devastating course as long as conditions are right for the *A. aegypti* vector and susceptibles remain in the human population. The case-fatality rate in such epidemics has been known to run as high as 70 per cent. Once established, the urban form of the disease becomes independent of the zoonotic reservoir but direct person-to-person spread does not occur, so the disease is limited to the geographic distribution of the Aedes vector.

Although yellow fever does not, at this time, present an epidemic threat outside the tropics and sub-tropics, a number of features of the disease merit more intensive examination.

Dengue fever

Dengue has long been familiar as a relatively mild if painful affliction of life in the tropics. Epidemiologically, the disease has been of particular interest since it is caused by a group B Arbovirus antigenically related to yellow fever virus and, like it, is principally transmitted through the human population by the mosquito vector, *A. aegypti*. It has been suspected that it may induce some cross-protection against yellow fever and that its endemicity in India and Southeastern Asia may account for the absence of yellow fever from those areas. The coexistence of the two diseases in Africa, however, has recently cast doubt upon that theory.

The dengue virus has recently developed a capacity for causing epidemics of haemorrhagic fever, especially among children under 14 years of age. The first such recent epidemic was in the Philippines in 1953[23, 24] when it caused over 750 cases with about 10 per cent fatalities. Since then some 500 cases a year have been admitted to hospital in the Philippines. This outbreak signalled the start of a spreading series of similar outbreaks across Southeast Asia. In Bangkok, Thailand, there were about 10,000 known cases between 1958 and 1965 with 698 deaths, all but 25 were children under 14 years of age. In 1973, Thailand recorded over 8,000 cases with 310 deaths while in Mandalay, Burma, haemorrhagic dengue first appeared in 1974 with 39 recognized cases and 17 deaths. This initial epidemic was followed in 1975 by 1,752 cases with 38 deaths, in 1976 by 954 cases with 27 deaths and in 1977 by 443 cases with 18 deaths.

The disease has several interesting and important features for the present study. First, the case-fatality rate in these haemorrhagic episodes has varied from about 3 per cent to about 7 per cent suggesting that enhanced virulence in a previously inoffensive virus. Second, the haemorrhagic syndrome is almost confined to indigenous children under 14 years of age. Caucasian children in the same epidemics have almost exclusively suffered from the classical clinical type of disease. Third, the haemorrhagic syndrome has so far been confined to the Far East and the Western Pacific Islands. It has not occurred in the Caribbean, although recently, the largest epidemics of dengue have been in that region. However, in 1977, an outbreak of classical dengue occurred in Jamaica and was found to be due to Type I of the four dengue serotypes – a serotype which is endemic and epidemic in the Far East and Africa but which has not previously occurred in the Caribbean. This event was followed in the same year by a Type II epidemic in Puerto Rico where 232 out of some 4,000 cases showed some bleeding tendency such as epistaxis, ecchymoses or low platelet count.

Although the occurrence of epidemics of haemorrhagic dengue appears to be a recent development in the disease, Halstead[23] has uncovered five previous reports showing that the virus has, for some years, been capable of producing haemorrhagic disease with shock and significant mortality. The first report was from North Queensland, Australia, in 1897 and the next four, from 1922–31, from the US, South Africa, Greece and Formosa.

The cause for the change in the clinical picture has not been determined but it has been suggested that it may be due to one of the following:

(1) a change in the intrinsic virulence of the virus itself;
(2) simultaneous infection with two dengue serotypes;
(3) a hypersensitivity reaction triggered by sequential infections with two different serotypes at a critical interval of time.

There does not appear to be strong evidence to support any of these three hypotheses.

Dengue virus is transmitted exclusively by mosquitos of which the most important is *A. aegypti*, and there is no record of person-to-person spread of infection. The distribution of the disease is, therefore, limited by its vectors.

Chikungunya fever

The name of this fever is derived from a local African word for the 'doubling-up' which arises from the excruciatingly painful arthritis which, in most cases, is the main symptom of the disease. The virus was first isolated from an epidemic in Tanzania in 1952–53, but has since been found to have a wide distribution. It has been isolated during epidemics in India and Southeast Asia as well as in East, West and Southern Africa.

The disease takes the form of a diphasic fever with excruciating joint pains and, during the second phase, a maculopapular rash frequently develops on the trunk and extensor surfaces of the limbs. Recovery is usually complete.

The virus is transmitted by *A. aegypti* and *A. africanus* in Africa and by *A. aegypti* and *A. albopictus* in India and Southeastern Asia. No vertebrate reservoir has been discovered but African monkeys are suspect. Person-to-person transmission has not been reported.

The association of Chikungunya fever with haemorrhagic manifestations is in some doubt since that clinical picture has not been observed in Africa and its occurrence in India and Southeastern Asia is complicated by the simultaneous presence of dengue fever which is known to produce haemorrhagic fever in that area.

The disease is not usually life-threatening and, in the absence of person-to-person spread, does not appear to present an epidemic threat to the developed world.

Rift Valley fever

Rift Valley fever was first recognized as a specific entity in 1931 in East Africa by Daubney *et al.*[26] who isolated the virus from sheep, cattle and human contact cases. From that time the disease has caused a number of very destructive epizootics in livestock in Eastern and Southern Africa with concomitant human cases, the majority have occurred as a result of direct contact with sick or dead animals. In South Africa there was a huge epizootic in 1951 where more than 100,000 sheep and cattle were estimated to have died and some 20,000 associated human cases occurred. In man, the virus caused a mild influenza-like illness and there were no fatalities despite the very large number of infections. However, two years later in 1953, a second epizootic occurred and this time, the associated human cases included a few where visual disturbances were noted – some leaving permanent sequaelae. As in the previous epidemic, transmission to man was mainly by direct contact with sick livestock, frequently involving autopsies which were carried out with bare hands. Remote infections were scarce and no person-to-person spread was seen.[29]

Following these two epizootics, the disease remained quiescent in this region until 1975 when a third major epizootic revealed a more sinister development. Seventeen severe human cases required hospitalization; four – all of whom died – exhibited the characteristics of haemorrhagic fever.[31] By this time, field studies [28, 29] had shown that primates, ruminants and rodents were all susceptible to infection but no vertebrate reservoirs had been discovered. It had also been shown that several mosquito species were capable of transmitting the infection but only *Aedes caballus* and *Culex theileri*[29] could be directly incriminated as active vectors.

The next development of significance epidemiologically was the sudden appearance of the disease in Egypt in 1977, 1,900 km north of Kenya.[30, 32] The disease was probably introduced from East Africa by the camel trade and caused an extensive epizootic among sheep, cattle, goats and camels. Of major significance, was that in this outbreak and its continuation in the following year, some 18,000 human cases occurred with 598 deaths in people not generally associated with livestock. For the first time in the known history of the disease, vector-borne transmission of the virus had been responsible for a human epidemic and the vector was identified as *Culex pipiens* which is abundant not only in Egypt, but also in Europe.

Rift Valley fever is still a relatively mild disease. Its development in less than 50 years during this century from an apparently new disease of livestock with limited human occupational incidence, emerging from an unknown reservoir to the status of a vector-borne human epidemic disease with significant mortality and a vector whose range extends into Europe, must be regarded with some disquiet.

Tick-borne and mite-borne group

Crimean-Congo haemorrhagic fever

During the summers of 1944–45 a new severe febrile disease occurred in the Steppe region of Western Crimea and caused over 200 cases, many among Soviet troops assisting with the grain harvest. Blood samples from acutely ill patients yielded a virus of the Flavivirus group and the same virus was isolated from ticks of the genus *Hyalomma*. As with many of the 'new' diseases, once it was studied, the disease was recognized as one which had been known in other parts of Russia for many years and its distribution was shown to include Bulgaria, Yugoslavia and the regions bordering the Caspian and Black Seas.

More recently, the 'Congo' virus, isolated in Africa in 1956 which was found to be widely distributed in East and West Africa, was shown to be identical with the Crimean strains, and an outbreak in Pakistan in 1976 was also found to be due to the same virus.

Serological surveys have indicated that a variety of small mammals act as the natural reservoir for the virus and domestic cattle, sheep, goats and camels may also be infected. These infections, however, appear to be symptom-free and man alone suffers clinical disease, underlining his status as an incidental host. Transmission is exclusively by the bite of infected ticks or by laboratory accident, and person-to-person spread does not occur.

Kyasanur Forest disease

Although the virus responsible for this haemorrhagic fever is now known to be widely distributed in India and many species of ticks are capable of transmitting it, human infections have only been reported from villages around Kyasanur Forest in Mysore State. The reason is not known, but it may be associated with recent agricultural extensions to the forest which have increased the exposure of domestic animals and the human population to infectious tick bites. Ticks are very abundant in the area and in 1957 it was noted that illness and death occurred in the forest monkeys before the appearance of human infections.

Infection occurs through the bite of infected ticks and there is no person-to-person spread.

Omsk haemorrhagic fever

Omsk haemorrhagic fever appeared as an epidemic disease in 1945 and 1948 in Siberia and is closely associated with muskrats in the swampy northern forest-steppe-lake region. Muskrats were only introduced into the area some 60 years ago and are presumably not the primary animal reservoir, which remains unidentified. The virus is, however, transmitted by ticks, and human infection can also occur by direct contact with muskrats. Person-to-person transmission does not occur.

Korean haemorrhagic fever with renal syndrome

This disease was first encountered by the Western world in 1951 as a severe epidemic haemorrhagic fever with renal involvement which affected troops in the Korean War. This disease was not new; it had already been recognized by Russian investigators in 1913, and in the 1930s an epidemic occurred in the Amur River basin between Siberia and Manchuria. A similar disease has now been reported from Scandinavia, Eastern Europe and Japan.

The virus has not been isolated in the laboratory, but the disease has been transmitted by inoculation of ground-up mites obtained from field mice in the epidemic zone. Person-to-person spread does not occur.

Rodent-associated group

Argentinian haemorrhagic fever

Argentinian haemorrhagic fever (AHF) was first encountered in epidemic form during the 1950s in the northwest region of the province of Buenos Aires. The disease is usually severe with few inapparent infections and 10–20 per cent of the cases with severe haemorrhagic manifestations culminate in death.

Between 1958 and 1974, almost 16,000 cases were notified on clinical grounds and experience since 1965 suggests that more than two-thirds of these could be virologically confirmed.

Although the disease is found only in a restricted area of some 100,000 km^2 out of the 3 million km^2 of Argentina, the endemo-epidemic area has expanded fivefold during the past 20 years and lies in the richest farming land of Argentina. Moreover, 50 per cent of the population lives either within the afflicted area or within 80 km (50 miles) of it.

The viral agent, Junin virus, belongs to the newly designated Arenavirus group[86] which includes Bolivian haemorrhagic fever virus, Lassa virus and lymphocytic choriomeningitis virus. These viruses all produce prolonged infections in rodents with persistent viraemia and viruria and are transmissible to man seemingly without the intervention of an arthropod vector although mites have been suspected in AHF.

The epidemiological features of the disease are instructive. First, although several species of two rodent families, Cricetidae and Muridae, coexist in the region only Cricetidae, represented by two species of the genus *Calomys*, appears to be capable of acting as an effective reservoir. *Mus musculus*, on the other hand, acts as a reservoir for lymphocytic chorio-meningitis virus and human infections, sometimes in the same individual, occur with both viruses. There is a marked seasonal incidence to the disease, the epidemic period coinciding with the period of rapid proliferation of the *Calomys* reservoir and culminating with the harvest during May. Infection is four times more common in males than in females and is more prevalent in rural workers than in the urban population. Clearly, close association with the field rodent reservoir is the key factor although the precise mode of transmission to man has not been determined. The virus shows no tendency towards person-to-person spread.

Despite the rapid expansion of the endemo-epidemic area and the threat which AHF poses to the population – particularly those in rural areas – the disease is tied closely to its restricted rodent reservoir and does not appear to constitute a world threat.

Bolivian haemorrhagic fever

The same conclusion may be reached for Bolivian haemorrhagic fever (BHF) which, both clinically and epidemiologically, is very similar to its Argentininan counterpart. First encountered in 1959, the disease has since caused regular epidemics in the affected area of Bolivia, the case-fatality rate reaching 30 per cent in one major epidemic.

The causative Machupo virus is also a member of the Arenaviruses and its reservoir is a third species of the same rodent genus, *Calomys callosus*, which is distributed through the plains of eastern Bolivia, northern Paraguay and the western fringes of the Mato Grosso State of Brazil. Machupo virus infected animals, however, are restricted to three areas in the Department of Beni in Bolivia. During epidemic periods this rodent is found in large numbers in the affected area and a high percentage of them are infected.

Despite the similarity of the disease to AHF, there are two significant differences. First, one episode of person-to-person transmission has been documented[42] where a case infected in Beni carried the infection to a neighbouring town and caused five secondary cases, four of which died. This episode appears to be unique and was presumably due to exceptional circumstances but is nonetheless disturbing. Second, the rodent reservoir, *Calomys callosus*, although primarily a field dweller, shows a marked predilection for human habitations and readily adopts a peridomestic way of life proliferating to a degree not seen in the absence of man.[41] In infected regions, this tendency greatly increases the risk to inhabitants of infested houses and removes the bias towards predominance of infection in adult male rural workers. It has further permitted the effective use of domestic rodent control techniques by trapping and poisoning as a means of preventing infections in village and urban communities.

Although successful in controlling and preventing human epidemic infection by eliminating domestic infestation with the rodent, these techniques do not, however, reduce either population or infection levels of *Calomys callosus* in the rural setting, and spread of enzootic infection with resulting expansion of the human endemo-epidemic region has occurred since the first appearance of the disease. Further extension of the infected area is clearly possible, and could occur, because of the distribution of the rodent.

Though neither the Argentinian nor the Bolivian haemorrhagic fevers would appear to constitute a world threat today, it does seem likely that their recognition in the 1950s was due to their initial appearance at that time rather than to the fact that they were old diseases which had previously escaped attention as was the case with the tick-borne fevers.

Lassa fever

Lassa fever was first encountered as a 'new' disease in an elderly American missionary nurse in Lassa, Nigeria, in 1969. This initial occurrence gave rise to a chain of infection involving two more missionary nurses and two laboratory scientists in the US. Since then, there have been over 380 recorded cases with over 100 deaths. The disease quickly gained notoriety for its extreme danger to hospital staff caring for sick patients and triggered public health reaction in a number of Western communities which feared the possibility of widespread lethal epidemics. Lassa fever will be considered in detail in Section Two.

Marburg disease

Marburg disease occurred simultaneously in three European localities in 1967 – Marburg, Frankfurt and Belgrade. All the primary cases were technicians involved in handling or establishing tissue cultures from one particular consignment of vervet monkeys from Uganda. There were 25 primary cases and 5 secondary cases occurred in their close contacts, four of whom nursed the original patients. A sixth, late secondary case occurred due to venereal transmission. This episode made a considerable impact in virological circles because, in addition to its suddenness, high mortality and unprecedented nosocomial (hospital) spread, the causative agent proved to be a 'new' virus of unique morphology. Despite the alarming transmission to people nursing the primary cases, there were no tertiary cases and no spread to the community at large.

The origin of the virus in Africa was not discovered and no further trace of the agent was encountered until 1975 when three cases occurred in Johannesburg; the index case may have been infected in Rhodesia. A closely related virus caused the outbreaks of Ebola fever in the Sudan and Zaire in 1976.

Ebola fever

Ebola fever, named after a river in Northern Zaire, appeared as a major epidemic almost simultaneously in south Sudan and in northeastern Zaire in July–September 1976. The case-fatality rates, 88 per cent in Zaire and 53 per cent in Sudan, were among the highest recorded for a virus infection and in common with Lassa fever shared an extreme transmissibility to persons, especially hospital staff who cared for the sick patients. In 1979, a further epidemic in south Sudan followed a similar pattern with a case-fatality rate of 67 per cent. Although the responsible virus is closely related to the Marburg virus, it is distinct from it. These epidemics were the most startling events of modern infectious disease epidemiology and will be considered in detail in Section Two.

'B Virus' infection

Herpes B virus, or *Herpes simiae*, is the simian equivalent of the human cold-sore virus, *Herpes simplex*. It produces trivial disease in monkeys, but a highly fatal neurotropic infection in man characterized by an ascending paralysis of the Landry type. The human disease was first encountered in 1934 following the bite of a 'normal' monkey. Only two cases were reported before the 1940s when the disease emerged as a serious occupational hazard among monkey handlers and laboratory workers preparing and using monkey kidney tissue cultures for the production of poliovirus vaccine. Fortunately, the human disease has remained rare despite the fact that the virus is regularly encountered as a latent infection in tissue cultures prepared from monkey kidneys, and the virus has shown no capacity for person-to-person spread. The disease appears to be without epidemic potential.

Bacterial diseases

Cholera

Cholera, together with smallpox, plague and yellow fever, make up the quartet of internationally notifiable, quarantinable diseases designated by the World Health Organization. The disease is primarily waterborne and has long been a scourge of populations in the Far East who live in conditions of minimal hygiene and grossly contaminated water supplies. At long intervals cholera has tended to develop pandemics which classically invade Europe from its Asian home both through its eastern land-trade routes and by sea. The spread is characteristically slow but relentless and is illustrated in Figure 1 which shows the progress of the latest pandemic starting from the Celebes in 1961.

This pandemic wave has engulfed India, the Middle East and large areas of Africa but has not progressed into Europe beyond Eastern Europe in the north and Spain and Portugal in the south. It has also failed to invade the New World countries of the Western Hemisphere, although a few isolated cases have occurred. In this respect the present pandemic differs from that of the early 1800s which reached Canada and the US in 1832 which was brought over, together with typhus and smallpox, by refugees from the Irish potato famine.

The disease has always afflicted primitive populations living in poor conditions of hygiene and has exacted its highest mortality from the poor and undernourished.

Transmission is exclusively by the oral route and is derived either directly or indirectly from contaminated water. It is unlikely in the extreme that epidemic spread could occur in prosperous, developed communities supplied with piped chlorinated water. At the worst, self-limiting outbreaks might occur in small isolated communities still dependent on septic tank or out-house sanitation and well or lake water. North American holiday camps and shooting and fishing lodges could be centres for such outbreaks.

Although the introduction of cholera into some areas of Central or South America could result in serious consequences, the disease does not constitute an epidemic menace to developed countries.

Legionnaires's disease

In July 1976, an explosive outbreak of pneumonia with high mortality which occurred in American Legionnaires attending a convention in Philadelphia, focused startled attention upon

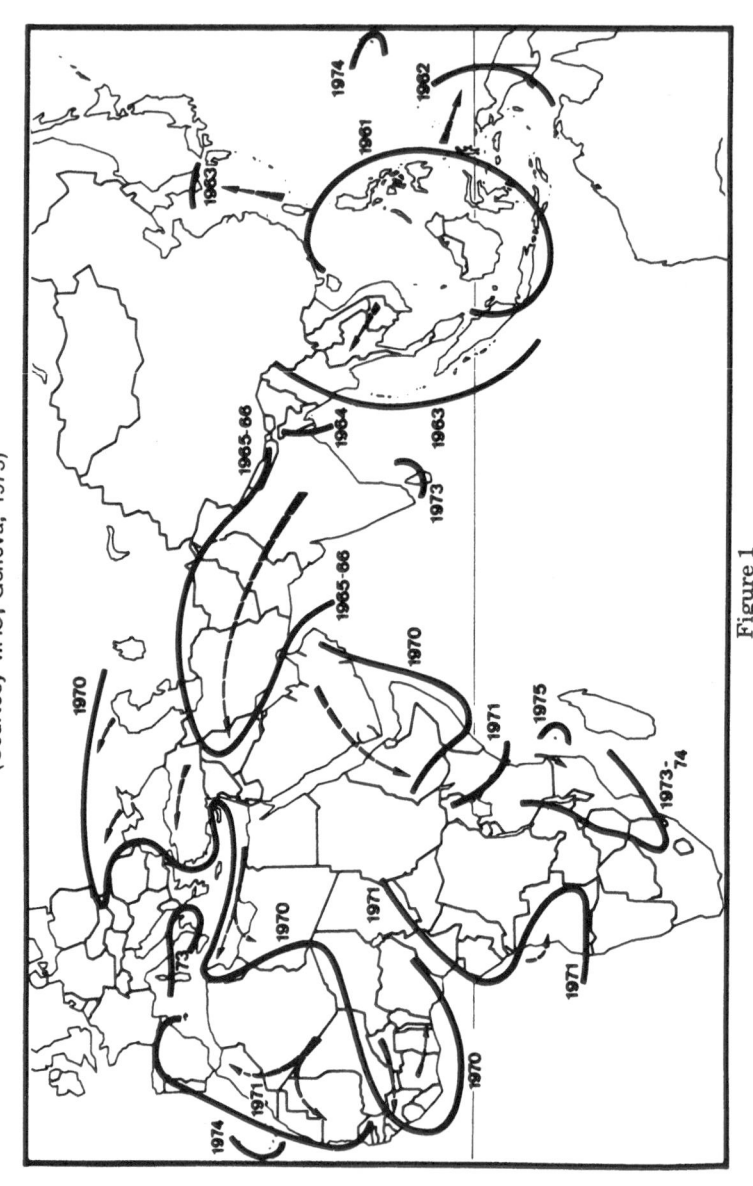

EXTENSION OF CHOLERA 1961-1975

(Courtesy WHO, Geneva, 1975)

Figure 1

an apparently new disease for which no immediate cause could be determined. The outbreak had a common source pattern with a total of 182 cases and 29 deaths but no evidence of secondary person-to-person spread of infection.

The epidemiology of the outbreak and the search for the causative agent was primarily conducted by the Center for Disease Control (CDC) in Atlanta, Georgia, in a classical major research programme and proved extremely difficult. It was not until January 1977 that the successful isolation of a causative bacterium could be announced. The progress of the investigation is fully reported in a series of reports from CDC and other investigating teams,[158] and the current state of knowledge in the proceedings of the International Symposium held at the CDC, Atlanta, in November 1978.

Isolation of the responsible organism now named *Legionella pneumophila*, permitted CDC to trace previous outbreaks of pneumonia which had no identifiable aetiological agent and to test patients' sera, stored and frozen against just such an eventuality, for the presence of antibodies against the newly discovered bacterium.

In this way, it was shown that the organism had been responsible for outbreaks as far back as 1965. Eickhoff[160] has reviewed 10 outbreaks, 4 preceding and 5 following the critical Legionnaires' episode in Philadelphia. During the three years following that outbreak in 1976, a total of 494 new sporadic cases were reported from 30 states across the US, and in 1978 and 1979 cases were reported originating in several European countries and Australia.

These investigations and widespread reports showed that the disease was, in fact, neither new nor confined to North America and that it usually occurred in sporadic form although outbreaks with the hallmarks of common-source infections have not been uncommon. These have varied from eight to 182 cases and the few attack-rates which have been calculable have been in the region of 1–5 per cent with the single remarkable exception of the 1968 episode in Pontiac, Michigan, where 144 infections occurred in a population at risk of 152 individuals – an attack rate of 95 per cent. This outbreak was also remarkable because the disease was mild and no fatalities occurred. In all other episodes, the case fatality rate has varied from 6–17 per cent in otherwise healthy individuals and from 29–53 per cent in patients with pre-existing disease such as renal failure, carcinomiatosis or comprised immunological status. The overall fatality rate in 558 cases associated with 10 outbreaks has been 14 per cent.

By November 1978, 494 sporadic cases had been reported from 63 states in the US in addition to confirmed outbreaks in 11 states. All outbreaks have been of the common-source variety and the organism has now been isolated from the environment, particularly from the water of air-conditioning cooling towers and evaporative condensers, in association with four outbreaks. There seems to be no doubt that the route of infection is respiratory with direct invasion via the lung and that air-conditioning systems constitute the usual vehicle of transfer to the human population. The true natural habitat of the organism remains in doubt and the first identified outbreak in St Elizabeth's Hospital, Washington, D.C., in 1965 suggested that the source of infection might have been soil excavations in the hospital grounds. It is clear that air-conditioning systems can be functioning only as an inanimate link, and probably an amplifying, reservoir, but technical difficulties arising from the very slow replication of the organism and its fastidious nutritional requirements for *in vitro* culture make the tracing of its ultimate environmental source extremely difficult.

Although much still remains to be learned about the distribution of the organism in nature and the epidemiology of the disease, it seems clear that it is exclusively a saprozoonosis, like coccidiomycosis and histoplasmosis, where human infection occurs directly from an environmental source. Of critical importance is that in all the outbreaks so far reported, diligent enquiry has failed to document a single instance of person-to-person spread of infection. Even in the hospital setting, outbreaks among patients have been due to common exposure; no evidence has been obtained to suggest that nursing Legionnaires' disease patients constitutes a danger to staff. Staff who have been involved in nosocomial outbreaks have themselves been exposed to the common source of infection.

Under these circumstances, the disease may present a serious local threat and in the future may well cause large common-source outbreaks, but it could not cause a spreading community epidemic and so may confidently be excluded from further detailed consideration in the present context.

Plague

Bubonic plague has been one of the greatest epidemic scourges of mankind from pre-Christian times to the present. Only since the demonstration of the zoonotic nature of the disease and the role of the black rat as the source of human infection has effective control been established. Since the work of the British Plague Commission in India, in 1905 and the ensuing years, has the epidemic form of the disease been virtually eliminated leaving a residue of enzootic infection in wild rodents in several areas of the world including the US.

These sylvatic reservoirs result in sporadic human infections which seldom progress to identifiable outbreaks since person-to-person transmission is rare and intolerance of rats prevents the massive build-up of rat populations in close association with man, at least in the more developed countries, which would permit flea-borne epizootics which could cause infection on an epidemic scale. It is therefore unlikely that a serious hazard of epidemic bubonic plague exists in developed communities.

The danger lies not with bubonic plague but with the pneumonic form of the disease which has a case-fatality rate approaching 100 per cent in untreated cases and has an awesome record of person-to-person transmissibility by the respiratory route. A few cases of plague occur every year in the US and the possible consequence of its introduction in its pneumonic form into a major city, in this instance New York, has been graphically told by Cravens and Marr.[144] This danger will be discussed in detail in Section Two.

Conclusions

From this preliminary examination of the candidate diseases it may be concluded that smallpox, yellow fever, Lassa, Marburg and Ebola fevers and plague might pose significant epidemic threats to developed communities. The rest may be excluded. Detailed discussion will, therefore, be limited to these six diseases.

Section Two

The Designated Diseases

4

Smallpox

Epidemiology

1. History and epidemic potential

Smallpox will be considered only briefly since the last known case anywhere in the world occurred in October 1977[4] and the disease was officially declared eradicated on 26 October 1979, an achievement of international collaboration unparalleled in history.

The disease shares with plague the distinction of being one of the most devastating scourges of mankind throughout history and its eradication has been a monumental feat of courage, determination and international cooperation under the World Health Organization. The story has been told by Dr Donald A. Henderson, the principal architect and driving force of the eradication campaign.[3, 4] Although it should now be possible to eliminate smallpox from consideration, few public health authorities would be prepared to do so for a few years to come. Therefore the disease will be discussed.

Smallpox is an ancient disease which dates back to prehistoric times. It emerged in Europe, probably from the Far East, around the sixth century AD and has remained endemic until the present century. It was introduced into the Americas by the Conquistadors and again by the early settlers in North America; it was re-introduced into Canada, along with cholera and typhus, at the time of the mass immigration which followed the Irish potato famines in the 1840s. It was not finally eliminated as an endemic disease from Europe or the US until about 1950.

Since the end of World War II, there have been numerous

importations of smallpox into Europe, especially the UK, the largest resulting outbreak was in Yugoslavia in 1972 when 175 cases occurred with 35 deaths. Canada and the US have largely escaped such importations although there was a major outbreak in New York in 1941, and a single case, a boy from Brazil, entered Canada in 1962 and reached Toronto before being diagnosed.

Before the WHO eradication programme in 1967, there were four major endemo/epidemic areas of smallpox in the world. Two, Indonesia and India, were afflicted with the classical Asian disease of *Variola major* with a case-fatality rate of about 40 per cent. South America was afflicted with the relatively avirulent *Variola minor* with a fatality rate of less than 2 per cent and Africa had a disease of intermediate severity with a 10–20 per cent fatality rate except in Ethiopia where the fatality rate was less than 1 per cent. In all, about 30 countries throughout the world reported one or more cases each month and the world incidence was about 131,000 cases per year. By the end of October 1977, the last known case of smallpox anywhere in the world had been reported.

This remarkable result had been achieved by applying diligent surveillance and extending the 'ring vaccination' procedure which can effectively control small individual outbreaks. This extension involved vaccinating the entire population in a zone surrounding the epidemic area and preventing travel out of it. This procedure, introduced in Nigeria by Dr Foege, now director of CDC, Atlanta, was so effective that it superseded the less reliable mass vaccination campaign and came to be known as 'surveillance-containment'.

The successful outcome of the smallpox eradication programme as compared with the disappointments encountered with yellow fever and malaria was due to certain characteristics of the virus and the disease which it causes.

(1) Man is the only known host in nature so there is no problem of animal reservoirs.
(2) Transmission is strictly person-to-person. Although it may be either direct or indirect through the inanimate environment, arthropod vectors are not involved.

(3) The disease is acute and easily detected and recognized, subclinical infections are rare, and there is no convalescent carrier state. There are, therefore, no hidden channels of infection in the community.

(4) A case does not become infectious until at least two days after the onset of illness by which time the patient is usually too ill to be ambulatory so community contacts are restricted in numbers.

(5) The disease has, with little variation, a two-week incubation period which is administratively convenient, giving time for contact tracing and establishing surveillance.

(6) Following recovery, immunity is solid and vaccination confers an almost equally solid, though less long-lived, immunity.

(7) There is only one antigenic type of the variola virus with no strain variation, so vaccination with vaccinia virus is universally effective.

(8) Vaccination of infected contacts during the early part of the incubation period confers protection. If carried out during the first four days, protection may be complete, while up to the sixth day, there is usually reduction in severity of the disease. Protection may be enhanced by injecting vaccinia-immune globulin.

The final characteristic (8), although of limited importance in the major eradication programme, is extremely important in the control and containment of small outbreaks. It is the basis of 'Ring Vaccination' where all traceable contacts are vaccinated as early as possible and placed under surveillance. This is followed by vaccinating all secondary contacts of the primary group. Protection can be enhanced by administering vaccinia-immune globulin. Selective vaccination on this model proved very effective in post-war Britain and avoided exposing large numbers of individuals to the hazards inherent in the vaccination procedure.

The main problem in the control and containment of smallpox lies in the exceptional stability of the virus both in aerosols and on inanimate objects. It may persist for years in dust or scabs derived from patients' skin lesions and is present in huge quantities in clothing or linen contaminated with serous or purulent exudates from the eruption. Massive secondary aerosols are easily derived from such materials and the virus, which is infective by the respiratory route may, due to its stability, be windborne for long distances without inactivation.[6] Out of a total of 71 cases in the 1961–62 epidemic in England and Wales, there were only four cases where no contact could be established and they all occurred within two miles of a smallpox hospital where active cases were being treated. These four cases gave rise to 48 secondary cases of which 18 died while the original introductions and their secondary cases numbered only 19 of which 8 died. The consequences of airborne spread within the hospital setting was later incontrovertibly shown in the Meschede incident in West Germany in 1970 when a single undiagnosed patient infected 17 persons on three hospital floors.[5]

These characteristics necessitate the most stringent structural and procedural isolation for the safe management of patients and for containment of the virus.

2. Case-fatality rate

There has been considerable variation in the case-fatality rate in different endemo-epidemic areas. Thus:

Variola major (Asia)	30–45 per cent
Variola major (Africa)	10–15 per cent
Variola minor (S. America and Ethiopia)	< 2 per cent

3. Community incidence

No figure can be given for community incidence. It has been extremely variable across the world and in different eras, and the disease has now been eradicated.

4. Seasonal incidence

While smallpox was widespread, its seasonal incidence tended to follow a constant pattern in any one region. The pattern varied greatly across the world since it was largely determined

by the population movements of migratory workers and pil-
grims.

5. Ecology

Because of its crucial implications for the eradication programme, the possible existence of an animal reservoir for
smallpox has received concentrated attention from the World
Health Organization. The search for any indication for such a
reservoir has been largely focused on West Africa and Zaire
since the last known case of smallpox in West Africa occurred in
1970 and in Zaire in 1971.

In 1975 an intensive surveillance programme was instituted
and 5 million schoolchildren in 12,000 primary schools, maternity child health centres and markets were examined by national and WHO teams looking for recent facial pock-marks which
had been found to be a sensitive indicator of past infection with
smallpox. No such marks were found which could be referred to
smallpox-like illness occurring after 1970 although many pock-
marks were found among older children who had been infected
prior to that year. In addition, a diligent search by 8,000 health
units failed to uncover any other indication of smallpox in any
of the countries involved. In Zaire, 16 smallpox surveillance
teams visit 4,000 health units throughout the country every six
months and during the five years to 1976, had collected over 500
specimens which were tested in collaborating laboratories in
Atlanta and Moscow. These studies failed to uncover any cases
of smallpox but did discover 12 cases of human monkey-pox
infection.[4, 8, 9]

The monkey-pox virus was first reported in 1959 in a captive
monkey colony in Denmark. Since that episode, nine similar
outbreaks have been reported in Europe and the US. The first
human case was discovered in Zaire in 1970 and 37 such cases
have now been reported, 28 from Zaire and the remainder from
West Africa. Six of the cases died. The disease is clinically
indistinguishable from smallpox, but the virus differs from the
variola virus both antigenically and in producing haemorrhagic
as opposed to white lesions on the chorioallantoic membrane of
developing chick embryos. The disease was of very low person-
to-person transmissibility even to intra-familial contacts and

such transmission was a possibility in only 2 of the 37 cases. The sources of the human infections have not been determined and ecological surveys have failed to reveal any animal reservoir even in the monkey population. Finding antibodies in a small proportion of monkeys may not be significant since the disease itself has never been observed in wild monkeys. Similarly, the finding of positive serology in other animal species is uninterpretable because of the cross-reactions seen within the pox-virus group.

The African surveys also led to the discovery in Moscow of another pox-virus; two strains of it were isolated from African monkey kidneys and two from the kidneys of wild rodents over a five-year period. This virus was indistinguishable from variola virus by any laboratory test.

In 1964 two strains of a similar virus were isolated in Utrecht from the kidneys of Malaysian cynomolgous monkeys. These six variola-like strains have been named 'white-pox virus' after the original Utrecht designation. Their infectivity for man is not known.[8, 9]

6. Vector requirements

Arthropod vectors are not involved in the transmission of smallpox.

7. Mechanisms of transmission of infection

The primary focus of infection in human smallpox has never been demonstrated but is presumed to be in the respiratory tract, and the ability of the virus to invade the body by this route has been demonstrated in both man and monkeys – in man inadvertently,[5] in monkeys in the laboratory.[6] The virus itself is extremely hardy and resistant to drying; it is shed in enormous quantities from the skin lesions of smallpox eruptions and can produce massive secondary aerosols when contaminated clothing, blankets or bedlinen is disturbed. The transmission of the disease by fomites, especially to laundry workers, is almost certainly due to inhalation of secondary aerosols.

The virus can also be introduced into the body by direct inoculation through the skin but this gives rise to a milder type of infection with a relatively low mortality and, before the days of Jennerian cowpox vaccination, was practised as a prophylactic measure termed 'variolation'.

8. Infectious period of the patient

An individual with smallpox becomes infectious only after the onset of clinical illness at the time of the first development of superficial lesions. The earliest shedding of virus is from lesions developing on the oro-pharyngeal mucosa, but as soon as the stage of vesiculation is reached, the massive shedding of virus from ruptured skin lesions enormously enhances infectivity. Healing of the skin lesions ultimately leads to 'crusting', with live virus embedded in the crusts where its infectivity may be preserved for years. The patient must be considered to be infectious until the last crust has separated – a process which may take several weeks if melon-seed type scabs are deeply embedded in the horny layers of skin on the soles of the feet or the palm of the hand.

The environs of the patient may remain infective for years if crusts and contaminated dust are not scrupulously removed and all surfaces disinfected.

9. Transmissibility

In view of the hardiness of variola virus its resistance to drying, aerosolization, and its invasion by the respiratory route, transmissibility of smallpox is surprisingly low. Where other viruses transmitted by the respiratory route, such as measles and influenza, will infect nearly all susceptibles in a family group, smallpox has been found to spread on average to fewer than 50 per cent even under relatively primitive and overcrowded conditions of family life – in spite of the fact that experimental work has shown that a single virus particle is probably capable of causing infection.[7] It is likely that this low degree of transmissibility is a reflection of the usually indirect spread of infection by secondary aerosols. At the same time, the extreme hardiness of the virus and its capacity for airborne transmission over long distances make it difficult to contain without extreme isolation precautions.

Biology

Identity

The variola virus is one of the *Poxviridae* whose members are the largest and most complex of the animal viruses. They have a distinct inner nucleoidal structure, lens-shaped lateral bodies and an outer membrane composed of interwoven helically wound lipoprotein strands. In 'shadowed' electron micrograph preparations, the virions show as brick-shaped particles of approximately $300 \times 250 \times 200$ nm. When stained, they are just at the resolution limit of light microscopy but are readily seen by dark-field illumination. The nucleoid contains deoxyribonucleic acid (DNA). RNA is not present.

Variola virus multiplies readily on the chorio-allantoic membrane of developing chick embryos giving yields of over 10^7 infective particles/g of tissue. It may also be cultured easily in chick-embryo or human tissue culture but with much lower yields of infective virus.

Because of its large size, the virus is easily manipulated in the laboratory and may be washed and concentrated by relatively low-speed centrifugation.

Stability

The virus is remarkably resistant to inactivation by drying and will remain viable in dust or on surfaces for long periods of time if protected from sunlight. In the dried crusts from skin lesions it will remain viable for years when stored in the dark, even at room temperature.

The virus is rapidly inactivated by heating to temperatures above 60°C and is susceptible to the action of formaldehyde, gluteraldehyde, sodium hypochlorite and the quaternary ammonium compounds.

Antigenic constitution

The antigenic constitution of variola virus is complex and there is a close antigenic relationship with other pox viruses notably cowpox and vaccinia viruses with which it shares a completely cross-protective antigen, the basis of protection against small-pox given by Jennerian vaccination. Each of these viruses exists only in a single antigenic type.

Mutability

Variola virus appears to be genetically stable as does vaccinia virus, but cowpox virus, which characteristically produces haemorrhagic lesions on the chorio-allantoic membrane of the developing chick embryo, tends to throw occasional non-haemorrhagic mutants which have been termed 'white variants'. These variants more closely resemble the non-haemorrhagic vaccinia virus and give some indication as to how this latter virus, which appears to be a laboratory artifact not found in nature, may have arisen.

In addition, genetic recombination among related pox-viruses is readily achieved by simultaneous infection of cells with two virus types. The virus progeny derived from the mixed genetic pool in infected cells take characteristics from both of the two parent strains. It is possible that vaccinia virus originated by accidental recombination of this type between variola and cow-pox viruses in the early days when cowpox was maintained by human arm-to-arm passage in the environs of smallpox hospitals.

The genetic stability of variola virus may be illusory despite the unchanging historical picture of smallpox since the disease recently existed in three different degrees of virulence characteristic of certain regions of the world. Genetically determined variation is certainly encountered in other pox-viruses.

Pathogenesis of infection

Portals of entry

The portal of entry of the virus in natural infection is almost certainly by the respiratory tract although the characteristic location of the primary lesion has never been established. It is thought to lie in the upper respiratory tract since primary pneumonia is an unusual feature of the disease.

Replication sites and spread through the body

The virus is capable of infecting any body tissue and, in the eruptive stage, is found to multiply in all deep organs as well as the skin. The virus is in fact pan-tropic rather than dermotropic although the skin eruption is the most clinically obvious feature of the disease.

Spread through the body is haematogenous and is thought to follow the mouse-pox model established by Fenner[1] in 1949. After initial multiplication in the primary focus, virus is carried to the regional lymph nodes where further multiplication occurs preceding spillover of virus into the blood to establish a primary viraemia. At this early stage the Kupfer cells of the liver and fixed macrophages of the spleen and bone-marrow effect a rapid clearance of virus from the blood and destroy many of the ingested particles as shown by the disappearance of viral antigen detectable by fluorescent antibody staining. Virus replication, however, becomes established in other cells and leads to a rapid build-up of virus terminating in a second spillover into the blood to produce a secondary viraemia.

The secondary viraemia probably marks the end of the incubation period and the onset of clinical disease as the virus generalizes and widespread replication begins throughout the body.

Distribution of virus

At the height of the disease virus is present not only in the blood and skin lesions but in all the organs and tissues with especially high concentrations in the liver, spleen, lung and adrenals.

Shedding from the body

Virus is shed from the body through the superficial lesions of the eruption. Consequently, the patient becomes infectious only with the development of a rash after clinical onset, the first shedding occurs from mucosal lesions in the oropharynx which ulcerate more rapidly than vesiculation occurs in the dermal lesions. Although virus is present in the skin lesions from their earliest stages, it is only with rupture of skin vesicles that massive shedding of virus begins. From this time, through the pustular stage until the lesions dry and crust, there is an outpouring of virus-laden exudate, usually blood-stained and purulent, which soaks into bedclothes and bedding producing gross environmental contamination. If such materials are permitted to dry, massive secondary aerosols may be generated by their disturbance.

The shedding decreases markedly with drying and crusting of the skin lesions but viable virus remains enclosed within the crusts so the patient cannot be regarded as non-infectious until the last crust has separated and the patient has dressed in clean, uncontaminated clothing after thorough bathing and superficial cleansing.

Because of the hardiness of the virus and its persistence in shed crusts and desquamated skin particles, contaminated fomites readily act as vehicles for transferring the infection (bedding and clothing are particularly dangerous to laundry workers). Viable virus may survive for years in room dust protected from sunlight.

Occasionally, patients may develop a primary variolous pneumonia at onset and are very infectious. Apart from this exceptional circumstance, however, smallpox is less infectious than might be expected from the disease picture and has been found to spread to fewer than half of the susceptible family contacts even under relatively primitive and overcrowded conditions.

Clinical factors

Prophylaxis

Successful vaccination with live vaccinia virus gives almost complete protection against infection for 2 to 5 years and protection against death from smallpox for 10 years or more. Individual immunity may be maintained at peak level by vaccination at 2–3 year intervals.

Vaccination of previously unvaccinated contacts during the first five days after exposure may afford complete protection from smallpox and even as late as the ninth day may modify the clinical severity of subsequent disease. Vaccination may be reinforced by the use of vaccinia-immune gamma-globulin. 'Marboran' (isatin-beta-thiosemicarbazone) has been shown to reduce the severity of the disease if given during the incubation period, but is relatively ineffective once the clinical disease has developed.

Treatment

There is no specific treatment. Antibiotics or chemotherapy in the eruptive stage is valuable in reducing the danger from secondary bacterial infection, but has done little to reduce the case-fatality rate. In severe cases, using sophisticated monitoring and life-support procedures would increase the danger of spread of infection and would contribute little to effective management.

Finally, it should be emphasized that the immunity afforded by successful vaccination is so effective that health-care personnel can be completely protected. Today, however, the proportion of hospital staff with up-to-date vaccinations is small and is dwindling.

5

Yellow Fever

Epidemiology

1. History

Yellow fever and smallpox are undoubtedly the oldest of the haemorrhagic fevers and with bubonic plague share the doubtful honour of being the most lethal killers among the great epidemic diseases. Just how old yellow fever is cannot be determined with certainty because of the difficulty in interpreting the early descriptions, written mostly by laymen, and because of the relative infrequency of travel, before the mid-fifteenth century, to those tropical regions where the disease was endemic. Scott in his *History of Tropical Medicine*[17] lists episodes as far back as 1493, but Blake[10] discounts many of these and considers that the earliest epidemic which can be reliably accepted as being what is now known as yellow fever is that of 1646–48 in Barbados, St Kitts and Yucatan, Mexico. Simpson[42] also accepts this date as the earliest authentic report.

Whether or not one accepts the earlier possible epidemics, it seems likely that a disease with the complex ecological background of yellow fever, which involves a monkey-mosquito-monkey sylvan cycle acting as a jungle reservoir, must be an ancient one even if its impact on major human populations through the derived man-mosquito-man urban cycle has only developed during the last 300 years.

Also uncertain is its place of origin. Although first recognized as a clinical entity in the Americas, there is good evidence that the disease has long been endemic in West Africa. Since the first European settlement in West Africa was established in 1482, while Christopher Columbus founded Ysabella in Espagnola (now Haiti) in 1493, 1,200 of its 1,500 founder members were dead by 1502, it is possible that the virus could have been transmitted in either direction. It seems, however, that the balance of evidence favours an African origin. The virus was introduced into the New World by trading vessels or imported slaves. The same vessels probably also introduced the mosquito vector *Aedes aegypti* which was able to breed freely in the bilges and water-butts of wooden ships and established itself in the West Indies, and then spread to the American mainland.

Whatever its origin, there is no doubt that, since the initiating epidemic of 1646–48 and the naming of the disease as 'yellow fever' by Griffith Hughes in 1750,[17] the main impact of the disease fell on the Americas to such an extent that its presence in Africa was not even suspected until the twentieth century and not verified until 1927 two years after the West Africa Yellow Fever Commission was established in 1925. Throughout the eighteenth and nineteenth centuries the virus and the disease were spread by ships, their crews and their mosquito-breeding bilges through the entire Caribbean area and along the coasts of America as far south as Ascension Island and Rio de Janeiro, and as far north as Halifax, Nova Scotia.

The epidemiological mechanism of this spread has been well documented in a series of striking episodes which were not understood at the time of their occurrence. The critical conditions for spreading the disease were: a susceptible crew, establishing *Aedes aegypti* in the ship with its breeding ground in the bilges and other collections of water, and the introduction of the virus either by shore-going sailors, shore-based labour or infected mosquitos which, once infective, remained so for life. With these conditions satisfied, a ship could maintain an active chain of infection as long as any crew member remained alive and uninfected and, when the last susceptible crew member had either died or recovered, thereby acquiring a solid immunity, infective mosquitos remained as a continued threat for weeks or months depending upon climatic conditions. In this manner, yellow fever was brought to British and European ports where the episodes remained clear-cut because of the absence of an indigenous vector to maintain the chain of infection.

In 1865 the *Hecla* sailed from Cuba and arrived in Swansea, South Wales, with a dying crew member on board. Following her arrival, customs officers and dock labourers contracted the disease and a total of 20 people who had anything to do with the ship were infected, including three members of the crew of a vessel moored alongside the *Hecla*. In the same year, the *Anne-Marie* reached St Nazaire from Havana after a six-week voyage. During the voyage, members of the crew were attacked by yellow fever and the last death occurred three weeks before her arrival. When her cargo of sugar was unloaded, many of the labourers developed yellow fever and members of the crews of seven vessels, which had moored for varying times close to the *Anne Marie*, were infected. These infections were certainly due to the presence of surviving infected mosquitos. Scott[17] lists 12 such introductions at Brest, St Nazaire, Swansea and Southampton between 1843 and 1867, and it is clear that in the American coastal trade such incidents must have occurred more frequently, depending upon the presence or absence of the *A. aegypti* and its density in the particular port.

Inevitably the disease followed the trade routes and the busier and more important the city the more frequently was it attacked. During the eighteenth century, the main brunt fell on Boston, New York and Philadelphia in the north and on Charleston, South Carolina, the only major city in the south at that time. After 1822, however, the disease virtually disappeared from the north and struck instead along the rapidly developing southern coastal cities from Charleston to New Orleans and Galvaston, Texas. The peak was reached with the New Orleans epidemic of 1853.[13] During the Civil War from 1861–65, the enforced quarantine of the southern ports by the northern blockade appeared to control the incidence of the disease. By the 1870s it was not only back but, with improved means of travel and a spread in the distribution of *A. aegypti*, it extended for the first time far up the Mississippi River, through Memphis, to St Louis, 1,000 km to the north and up the Tennessee River to Chatanooga, a distance of 600 km. The last epidemic of this final era was in 1905 when New Orleans was again attacked. By this time, Walter Reed's team had established the role of the mosquito in the transmission cycle and the epidemic was effectively nipped in the bud by vigorous mosquito control measures.

During this same period there were repeated introductions of the disease into the Caribbean Islands, most of which were too small to provide an adequate reservoir for maintenance of the virus, and also a spread of infection to the northern coasts of South America including Venezuela, Ecuador, the Guyanas, Surinam and Brazil. It must have been at this time that the virus entered the South American monkey population and the New World Sylvan yellow fever reservoir was established.

During these same two centuries the West African endemic areas must have been active and yellow fever was repeatedly introduced into Spain and less frequently into other Mediterranean countries. This activity must have been forgotten in later years since one of the terms of reference of the West African Yellow Fever Commission of 1925 was to determine whether the disease existed in West Africa.[21]

The total mortality caused by yellow fever during the seventeenth, eighteenth and nineteenth centuries must have been enormous. With the lack of any understanding of the aetiology of infectious disease generally, the erratic incidence of a vector-borne disease must have been utterly bewildering and it is not surprising that its contagious nature was hotly disputed. The only factor which was universally effective in controlling an epidemic was a drop in temperature – a climatic factor which had important, though unsuspected, implications since it ensured the annual total eradication of the disease from northern ports where winters were too cold for survival and subsequent breeding of the Aedes vector. In these ports, yellow fever was an exclusively summer disease and was eventually eliminated in the early nineteenth century when local boards of health enforced rigid quarantine procedures for arriving ships. In the South, such measures were much less effective.

Although the virulence of the virus in different epidemics appeared to vary, both the attack rate (often exceeding 30 per cent) and case-fatality rate (sometimes as high as 70 per cent) were usually high. In the Philadelphia epidemic of 1793, the entire city was brought to a virtual standstill with 17,000 cases and over 5,000 deaths in a population of about 40,000.[10] The epidemic in Memphis in 1878 was equally severe with some 15,000 cases and 3,500 deaths in a population of 35,000. In both these cities, there was a total disruption of normal life while the epidemic lasted and all who were able to fled to the country. It is interesting to contrast this impact with that of the 1853 epidemic in New Orleans when the medical profession, city council and newspapers managed, for commercial reasons, to deny the very existence of an epidemic until the yellow fever deaths exceeded 200 a day. Nevertheless, the population was reduced from over 200,000 to about 100,000 by a mass exodus which included most members of the city council. By the time cooler weather controlled the epidemic, some 9,000 deaths had been recorded, with the peak reaching 1,628 deaths in one week during the month of August.[13] As Duffy[13] points out, the development of the southern cities continued despite the repeated onslaughts of yellow fever – and other infections such as cholera – with not only rapidly expanding commerce but also rapidly increasing populations nurtured by the continuous arrival of immigrants and travellers undeterred by the ever-present threat of the disease. It is also interesting to contrast this philosophical acceptance of the danger of death by disease with the instant reaction of fear aroused by Lassa fever today.

Developments after 1900

In 1900 the entire situation dramatically changed. Up to that time, the cause of yellow fever was unknown and there was no agreement as to whether the disease was communicable. As Andrew Warren said:

> For more than 200 years yellow fever was one of the great plagues of the world. The tropical and subtropical regions of America were subject to devastating epidemics, while serious outbreaks occurred as far north as Boston and as far away from the endemic centers as Spain, France, England, and Italy. During this period appalling epidemics swept repeatedly over the West Indies, Central America, and the southern US, decimating populations, paralyzing industry and trade, and holding the people of these regions in a state of perpetual dread.[21]

In July 1900, however, Major Walter Reed was appointed president of a US Army Yellow Fever Commission and sent to Cuba where there was an epidemic. With the help of Dr Carlos

Finlay, a local Scottish physician who already suggested the role of the mosquito in transmitting the disease, Reed and his colleagues quickly proved that the disease was transmitted by mosquitos which became infected by feeding upon patients during the first three days of their fever and that the mosquitos required an incubation period of about 12 days before they became infectious.

Acting promptly upon this information, Major William Gorgas, chief sanitary officer in Havana, instituted anti-mosquito measures and by September 1901, had eradicated yellow fever from the city although it had been there in endemic and epidemic form for the past 150 years. In 1903, Cruz eradicated the disease from Rio de Janeiro by similar methods, and in 1904 Gorgas repeated his Havana success in Panama.

During the next 10 years, yellow fever was eliminated from most of the tropical ports of the Americas and in 1916 the Rockefeller Foundation Yellow Fever Commission instituted a programme for the world eradication of the disease responding to fears that opening the Panama Canal might introduce the infection to the Far East.

At the time, total eradication seemed a perfectly feasible goal. A preliminary survey had suggested that there were only a few endemic foci remaining in the Americas which were thought to comprise the only region in the world where the disease existed. The *A. aegypti* mosquito was the only known vector, and its peridomestic breeding habits made it relatively easy to control as Gorgas had demonstrated. If the endemic sources could be eliminated, the disease should be eradicated.

For a while the programme progressed well, but during the early 1930s things began to go wrong. First, it was found that mosquitos other than *A. aegypti* could transmit the disease and could even mediate urban epidemics; then yellow fever, usually as individual infections or small outbreaks, occurred in places where the disease was not known to be endemic or where it had already been eradicated. Increasingly these outbreaks were observed in the absence of *A. aegypti*. Next, five wild monkeys were found to possess antibodies against yellow fever – an event which had already been foreshadowed as early as 1914 when an epidemic in Venezuela had been preceded by an epizootic causing deaths in red howler monkeys.

From these episodes, and later from the examination of liver specimens taken by viscerotome from cases of unexplained deaths, it became apparent that a totally unsuspected yellow fever cycle existed in the jungle with a reservoir other than man and a vector other than *A. aegypti.* This 'sylvan' yellow fever was eventually shown to be an infection of forest monkeys living in the high jungle canopy and mediated by canopy mosquito vectors of the *Haemagogus* and *Sabethes* genera which rarely bite man except when disturbed. Later studies in Africa showed a similar cycle to exist among its forest monkeys, the main vector here is the canopy mosquito *Aedes africanus.* These sylvan cycles are independent of man, who becomes involved only as an incidental host, but they may initiate urban man-mosquito-man epidemics typically mediated by *A. aegypti.* In Africa, this association has been well delineated. The primary monkey cycle is mediated by *A. africanus* which lives in the forest canopy and bites after dark when the monkeys are asleep in their treetop resting places. *A. africanus* rarely bites man at ground level. Man becomes involved when monkeys forage in cultivated areas at the forest fringes where the semi-domestic mosquito *Aedes simpsoni* acts as a link vector. Field labourers so infected may then introduce the infection into *Aedes aegypti*-infested urban areas and institute a man-mosquito-man epidemic.[14]

With the elucidation of these cycles, surveys of the disease, based on serum neutralization tests and virus isolations from wild-caught mosquitos have been instituted, and on both sides of the Atlantic extension of previously known endemic areas has become evident. In South America, this has been to the southeast to reach the northern limits of Argentina and Paraguay and in Africa east to Ethiopia and Uganda (see Figures 2 and 3).

The evidence of activity is not entirely due to uncovering previously unsuspected endemic areas, for example, the Sudan-Ethiopia outbreak of 1959–62 in a region where no previous yellow fever had been known to occur. In Ethiopia, the case-fatality rate was 85 per cent in the most severely affected area and not less than 15,000 deaths were estimated to have occurred. A serological survey had been carried out in the area in 1955 but had revealed no yellow fever antibodies in the Akobo

NOTIFIED CASES OF YELLOW FEVER IN THE AMERICAS, 1950–1969 *

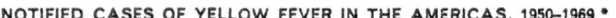

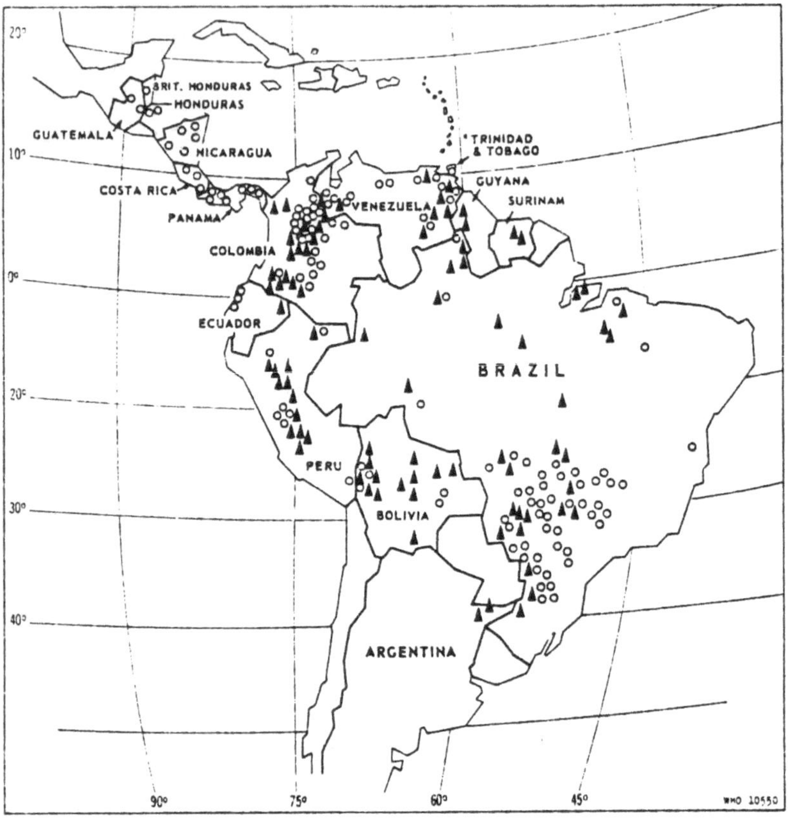

* Each circle or triangle represents one or more cases.

    o   1950–1959

    ▲   1960–1969

Sources: World Health Organization Expert Committee on Yellow Fever, 3rd Report 1971.
World Health Organization Technical Report Series **479**/1–56 (p. 9).

Figure 2

river valley where a 16 per cent positivity rate was found in 1961. At this time, 96 per cent and 92 per cent seropositivity were found in the Gilo and Baru river valleys, by which infec-

NOTIFIED CASES OF YELLOW FEVER IN AFRICA, 1950–1969 *

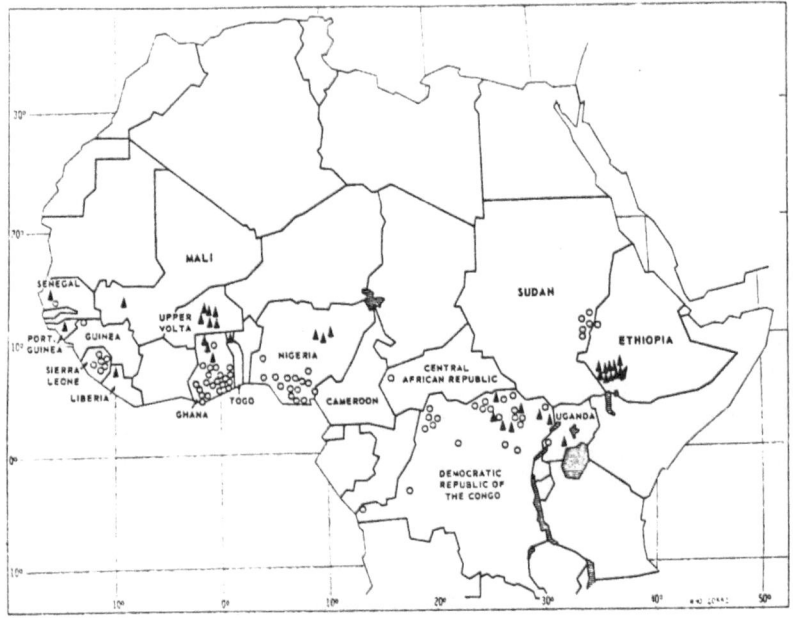

* Each circle or triangle represents one or more cases.

○ 1950–1959

▲ 1960–1969

Sources: World Health Organization Expert Committee on Yellow Fever, 3rd Report 1971.
World Health Organization Technical Report Series **479**/1–56 (p. 10).

Figure 3

tion must have reached the epidemic area southwest of the Blue Nile (see Figure 4).[18, 22] Similarly, in Bwamba, 48 of 275 individuals who were seronegative in 1939–40 were found to have converted to seropositive by June 1941. In the endemic area of West Africa, epidemic activity has occurred in Senegal in 1965 and in Nigeria in 1950–53 and 1969.[11] The last epidemic was estimated to have caused about 100,000 cases.[11] Zaire has been continually affected from 1950–61.

In South America the opening up of jungle hinterland, largely in connection with oil exploration, has caused a steady

YELLOW FEVER IN ETHIOPIA (1962)

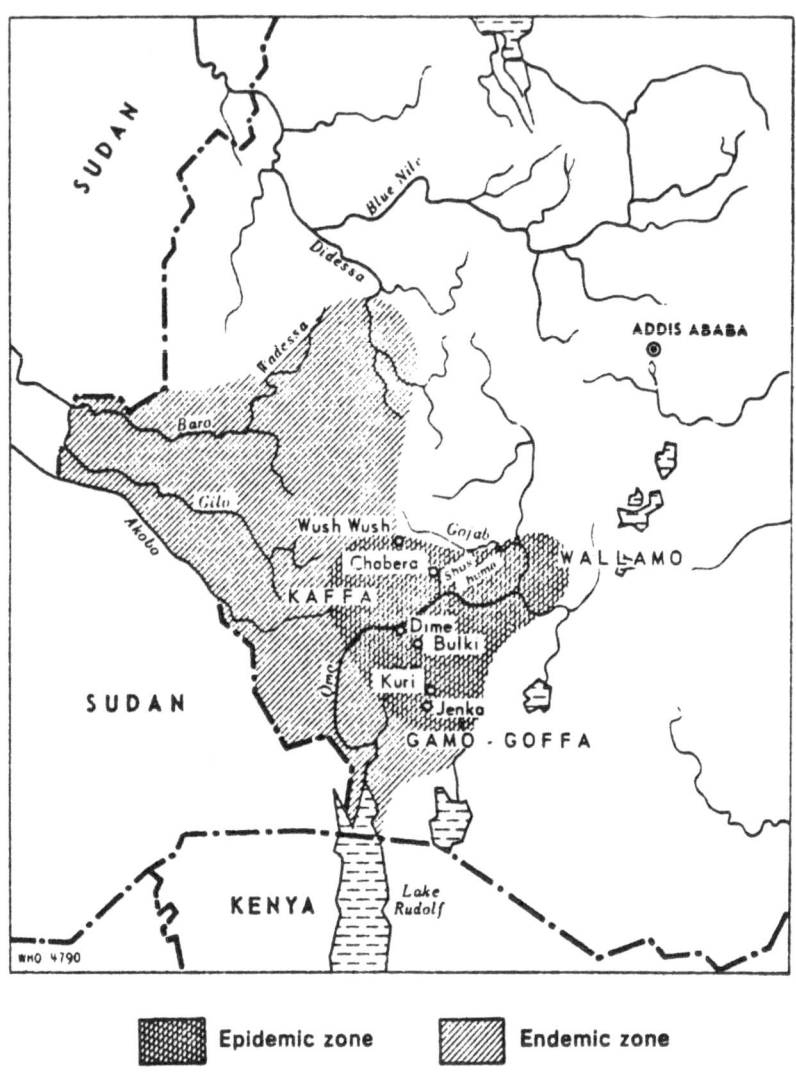

Source: World Health Organization Chronicle 1964. 18/390–392 (p. 391).

Figure 4

series of cases especially in Bolivia, Brazil and Colombia. Argentina had an outbreak in the north in 1965–67 and Peru has had a fairly steady incidence since 1950. In 1945, the virus reappeared in western Panama and spread through Central America as far as Mexico.

The disease was also reintroduced into Trinidad in 1954 with 15 human cases and four deaths and an epidemic among monkeys.

Present understanding of the epidemiology of yellow fever. The discovery of jungle – 'sylvan' – yellow fever destroyed the simplistic concept of the disease as an urban man-mosquito-man cycle with *A. aegypti* as the sole vector and also destroyed all hope of its world eradication. It is now evident that the maintenance reservoir for the virus lives in the forest canopy monkey-mosquito cycle with several species of both vertebrate host and vector involved. It is also possible that other primates may act as maintenance reservoirs since bush-babies (Galago spp.) are susceptible. It is even possible that the monkey cycle is itself secondary to a primary cycle in other animals which has never been discovered.

The fact that monkeys are very susceptible and suffer a high-case fatality, at least in the New World species, suggests that the disease is a relatively recent one to them. The human disease cycle is clearly incidental and the man-*A. aegypti* cycle is not usually capable of maintaining the disease indefinitely, largely because the infection results in a solid lifelong acquired immunity in survivors and the rapid spread of infection under epidemic conditions quickly exhausts the supply of susceptibles.

Since there is no human carrier state and the viraemic stage in cases of the disease is limited to three days, survival of the virus is wholly dependent upon the 'extrinsic' mosquito phase of the infection. The Aedes, once infected, remains infectious for life but does not transmit the virus trans-ovarially to subsequent generations. The lifespan of the adult is usually only a few months and after this the disease will die out unless fresh human susceptibles are found from which another generation of mosquitos can become infected. These factors combine with the high case-fatality rate to make the disease a dramatic epidemic pestilence which seldom achieves true endemic status in man.

The same factors also operate in the monkey cycle except that the canopy mosquitos may be carried for considerable distances by wind currents. Surviving monkeys also develop a solid lifelong immunity. In an epizootic area the great majority are likely to be infected so that here too the susceptibles in a given band will rapidly become exhausted. However, since monkeys are shorter lived and faster breeding than humans, this deficiency is more rapidly rectified. In the vast tropical jungles of Africa and South America the infection can travel continuously through the monkey population leaving behind it immune survivors to build a fresh susceptible population within a few years. Where the forests are smaller, as in the Caribbean Islands, the supply of susceptibles may be too small for even the monkey cycle to be maintained and the disease then dies out until reintroduced – an event repeatedly seen in the Americas and illustrated by the 1949 reintroduction of yellow fever into western Panama. It progressed westwards through Costa Rica, Honduras and Guatemala to Mexico where it died out in 1956 because it was unable to return through the narrow isthmus of its advance since a barrier zone of immunity followed it.

The corollary to this epidemiological balance is that, failing reintroduction of the infection, any community, whether human or monkey, will lose its immune status within a few generations and this has undoubtedly happened in the entire Caribbean area and in the human population of coastal North America. Where the *A. aegypti* is present in adequate density, this may develop into a potentially dangerous situation. This mosquito has been permitted to reinstate itself in many areas since the menace of yellow fever was removed and has recently shown itself capable of orchestrating impressive epidemics of dengue fever in the Caribbean area and along the north coast of South America. Dengue and yellow fever coexist in Nigeria and yellow fever has been proven to occur in patients with pre-existing antibody to Group B arbovirus[20] so the presence of dengue in an area can no longer be regarded as a safeguard against yellow fever. The Caribbean area, together with much of Venezuela and possibly Brazil, and some of the southern United States (where a programme to control *A. aegypti* was initiated in 1966 and abandoned in 1969 for lack of funds) must now be regarded as possible 'receptive areas' (see Figure 2, p. 54).

It is, however, to vast areas of India and Southeast Asia that this term most significantly applies. The building of the Panama Canal first raised fears of introducing yellow fever into the Far East and led the Rockefeller Foundation to begin a programme of total eradication. Although the ultimate goal could not be reached, the eradication of human urban yellow fever was achieved and the threat of the disease was largely removed. Despite this, the freedom of the Far East from yellow fever has never been satisfactorily explained in view of the wide distribution and high density of the vector, *A. aegypti*. The Asian strains of this mosquito have been shown to be perfectly capable of transmitting the disease; the rhesus monkey is highly susceptible, and it is now known that endemic dengue is not a protection from infection although the possession of Group B antibodies may modify the clinical course of the disease in individual cases. Epidemiologically, it would seem that the only protection is because yellow fever has never reached the east coast of Africa where trading vessels could have transported it to Asia as they probably did to America. If this is the case, then the continued protection of that region is very finely balanced and could be destroyed by the transportation by air of a single human case in the incubation period of the disease or of a single infected mosquito.

Clinical aspects

The classical clinical picture of yellow fever is of a biphasic fever of sudden onset with pronounced headache and backache. Jaundice is present in more than half the cases but may be confined to yellowing of the sclerae. Nausea and vomiting are frequent and, in severe cases, gastric haemorrhage leads to the famous 'black vomit' associated with the disease. In such cases haemorrhage may also occur from other body orifices.

After three days of high fever and extreme malaise a brief remission occurs when the fever abates and the patient's subjective condition improves. This phase may then blend into convalescence, but is more usually succeeded by a recrudescence of fever with clinical deterioration which may culminate in death at any time from the fifth day onwards. The white blood count shows an early leukopaemia frequently followed by leukocytosis especially in severe cases.

Recovery, when it occurs, is complete and no chronic infections or carrier states have been observed. Antibody is detectable in the blood from about the fifth day of illness and recovery is accompanied by a solid, lifelong immunity.

Around this median clinical picture the disease varies from subclinical infection, through mild infections without apparent jaundice to malignant and fulminant forms of the disease with severe haemorrhage and death as early as the third day.

Although the classical case may be diagnosed clinically with some confidence under appropriate circumstances, milder cases frequently cannot be diagnosed without the use of laboratory tests even during epidemic prevalences.

2. Case-fatality rate

Historically, yellow fever has been feared for its shattering epidemics and high mortality, and as recently as 1961 a case-fatality rate of 85 per cent was reported for the worst-affected area in the Ethiopian epidemic. In the great epidemics in the North American cities during the nineteenth century, reported case-fatality rates were usually between 20–30 per cent. In 1969 in Nigeria, the fatality rate among hospitalized cases was 40 per cent.[11]

It is clear, however, that these high estimates of fatality rates do not take mild, clinically undiagnosable and subclinical infections into account. By analogy with the recent findings in Lassa fever and by extrapolation from antibody surveys, it seems more likely that the infection-fatality rate is below 5 per cent in endemic areas although among frank cases it may well be around 20–30 per cent, and may be even higher under epidemic conditions. In the laboratory, considerable variations in virulence for animals have been observed in different virus isolates but it has not proved possible to correlate these laboratory studies with virulence in man.

3. Community incidence

The incidence of yellow fever is very variable in the endemic regions and has a strong occupational element. The sylvan cycle was discovered as a result of sporadic cases occurring among wood-cutters working in jungle areas. Oil exploration in the more remote regions of northern South America has given rise to increased exposure and numerous resulting cases in many areas. Under epidemic conditions, the incidence may rise to 30 per cent.

4. Seasonal incidence

Seasonal variation in incidence is significant only in fringe areas of the sub-tropics where low winter temperatures discourage or kill mosquito vectors. During the nineteenth century, the onset of cold weather in the autumn of the year was the only effective controlling factor in the North American epidemics.

5. Ecology

In its present form, yellow fever is almost exclusively a zoonosis maintained in monkey reservoirs and transmitted by a variety of forest mosquitos occupying the high jungle canopy which is the principal habitat of the monkeys.

The species of both monkeys and mosquitos involved in the maintenance and transmission of the virus in the wild differ in the two great natural endemic areas. In South America, the principal reservoirs are species of the Cebus, Ateles and Alouatta genera and transmission is chiefly by mosquitos of the *Haemagogus* and *Sabethes* genera. Mosquitos of both these genera may bite man in jungle surroundings especially when disturbed by tree-felling.

In Africa, the *Cercopithecus* and *Colubus* genera of monkeys form the main reservoir although other primates such as bush babies (Galagos spp.) may be involved. *A. africanus* appears to be the most significant vector in the sylvan cycle with *A. simpsoni* acting as a link vector to man. *A. simpsoni* was probably the vector responsible for the extensive Ethiopian and Nigerian epidemics.

6. Vector requirements

Yellow fever is exclusively transmitted by mosquitos which are infected by biting human or monkey hosts in the viraemic stage of their disease. In the mosquito, the virus derived from the ingested viraemic blood establishes an active infection which usually becomes fully established in 10–12 days but may take longer in cooler weather. The mosquito is not able to transmit the disease until its infection is fully developed and this delay has been termed the 'extrinsic incubation period'. The virus does no harm to the mosquito and once the mosquito becomes infectious, it remains so for life – which may be a matter of several months under favourable circumstances. During this period, it may bite every two or three days. Transovarial transmission is not thought to occur.

Many species of mosquitos have been shown to be capable of transmitting the virus. Haemagogus and Sabethes species are mainly involved in South America, while Aedes species, especially *A. africanus* and *A. simpsoni*, are the principal vectors in Africa. On both continents, urban yellow fever was transmitted almost exclusively by *A. aegypti* and such transmission still occasionally occurs though usually only on a household scale.

7. Mechanism of transmission of infection

The natural mechanism of infection transmission is by direct inoculation of the virus into the bloodstream by the bite of an infected mosquito which has completed the extrinsic incubation period needed for ingested virus to become established in the salivary glands. Walter Reed's original experiments demonstrated that there was no other natural mechanism of transmission and specifically, that close contact with sick persons and even wearing and sleeping in clothes and bedding soiled with the excreta and vomitus of yellow fever cases failed to transmit the disease. Transmission by laboratory accident has, however, occurred on many occasions and transmission by artifically generated aerosols has been demonstrated in the laboratory although person-to-person transmission by the respiratory route does not occur in nature.

8. Infectious period of patient and transmissibility

A case of yellow fever becomes infectious with the onset of illness after the intrinsic incubation period which may last from

3 to 10 days. The infectious state coincides with the onset of viraemia which lasts for no more than three days during the initial febrile stage of the disease. Female mosquitos feeding on the patient during this period ingest the virus and become infectious after the extrinsic incubation period.

Person-to-person transmission does not occur in the absence of the mosquito vector.

Biology

Identity

The causative agent is an arbovirus of antigenic Group B and is the type species of the genus *Flavivirus* which includes a range of mosquito-borne viruses including dengue and a number of other viruses causing viral haemorrhagic fevers (Table 1, p. 9).

The virus is small with a diameter of 30 nm, and has a lipoprotein envelope, which renders it sensitive to inactivation by lipid solvents such as ether and sodium deoxycholate. The viral nucleic acid is ribonucleic acid (RNA). The virus agglutinates the erythrocytes of certain species of birds, providing the basis for antibody measurement by haemagglutination inhibition.

Stability

The virus is extremely unstable even in aqueous suspension and is readily inactivated by standard disinfectants.

Antigenic constitution and relationships

There is only one antigenic type of the yellow fever virus and this has apparently remained stable over the years. Virus neutralization tests performed either in chick embryos or by intracerebral inoculation in mice are highly specific and may even detect minor strain differences within the species. However, by complement fixation and haemagglutination inhibition, cross-reactions occur with other arboviruses. These cross-reactions have formed the basis of antigenic classification and the major group to which yellow fever virus belongs has been designated as Group B. Within this group, the most important cross-reaction is that with the dengue virus since it has been thought that antibodies against the latter may confer some protection against yellow fever infection and therefore may account for the absence of yellow fever from Southeast Asia where dengue infection is rife. However, the demonstration by Spence *et al.*[20] of the occurrence of yellow fever in two patients who had pre-existing antibodies against the Group B arboviruses, presumably as a result of dengue infection in the Caribbean, has cast doubt upon this theory.

Mutability

The yellow fever virus appears to be genetically stable in that there is little variability in the clinical disease or the antigenic constitution of the virus in different regions, nor does the clinical picture seem to have varied during the last three centuries. Nevertheless, the virulence of different strains isolated in the wild shows considerable variation.

Clear evidence of selective adaptations is seen in the establishment of the two widely used vaccine strains of virus, Max Theiler's 17D strain, derived by prolonged passage in chick embryo tissue culture from which the central nervous system had been removed, and the French neurotropic strain developed by mouse intracerebral passage. Both strains were derived from virulent wild strains, the French vaccine strain losing its viscerotropism and the 17D strain losing both viscerotropism and neurotropism while retaining antigenicity. Both strains became modified to the extent that they could be used as live vaccines. The virus has never shown any tendency to vary towards enhanced virulence in man or direct person-to-person spread.

Pathogenesis of infection

Portals of entry

The only portal of entry in the natural disease is by transcutaneous injection directly into the bloodstream by the bite of an infectious mosquito.

Replication sites

Yellow fever is a pan-tropic infection in that the virus is generalized as a result of the early viraemia but the principal pathology lies in the liver and kidneys suggesting that these organs are the primary site of viral replication. The myocardium, however, is also affected and the haemorrhagic diathesis suggests that the vascular endothelium is also a site of viral multiplication. The central nervous system is not usually involved.

Spread and distribution

Spread through the body occurs via the blood during the stage of viraemia and leads to generalized distribution of virus.

Shedding from the body

Shedding of virus from the body does not usually occur in the natural illness. Viraemia is of short duration being confined to the first three days of illness, the stage of 'infection', during which the patient is febrile and may suffer from severe headaches and vomiting but haemorrhages do not occur. In the classical progression, this stage is followed by remission with a fall of temperature, disappearance of viraemia and subjective improvement in the patient. It is only in the third stage of 'intoxication' that haemorrhages occur accompanied by jaundice and severe renal involvement. At this time the classical 'black vomit' also occurs. Since viraemia has by now disappeared and free antibody is detectable in the blood, neither the vomit nor the frank haemorrhages are infectious.

Clinical factors

Prophylaxis

The Theiler 17D vaccine is probably the safest and most effective vaccine ever developed against an infectious disease. It is a live vaccine developed in cultures of chick embryo tissue where the central nervous system has been removed and is of minimal neuro- and viscero-tropism while retaining full protective antigenicity. It may be administered by scratch or by subcutaneous inoculation. The scratch is cheap and useful particularly for mass vaccination programmes while subcutaneous inoculation is preferable for individual vaccinations or for small groups. In early days, the inclusion of human serum as a stabilizing agent in the vaccine caused the inadvertent administration of Hepatitis B virus in a number of instances and led to the first recognition of 'serum hepatitis' as an infective entity. This complication caused much concern that the vaccine strain of virus was causing the jaundice in these cases. Once the true reason was recognized and human serum was eliminated from the preparation, the vaccine has proved to be extremely safe and effective.

The French neurotropic vaccine is also effective but causes occasional encephalitis. In the early 1960s, its use in Senegal was abandoned for this reason and a severe epidemic of yellow fever occurred in 1965.

Therapy and management

There is no specific therapy for the disease and management is limited to general supportive measures.

6

Lassa Fever

Epidemiology

1. History and analysis of outbreaks

Lassa fever appeared with dramatic suddenness in January 1969, as a lethal, previously unknown disease, which afflicted a missionary nurse in Lassa, Nigeria. It initiated a chain of infections involving two nurses who cared for the first case in the Bingham Hospital at Jos where she died, and extended to two laboratory workers in the US.

The first two cases died. The third barely survived after being flown to New York. The fourth survived only as a result of an immune plasma transfusion donated by the surviving third case, and the fifth case died.

Thus it was only by the narrowest margin that the virus failed to achieve a clean sweep with 100 per cent fatality in the first five cases it had ever been known to cause. The world was then faced with the eruption of an apparently new disease of unprecedented transmissibility and lethality. The drama of its first appearance was not lessened by a second outbreak at the Evangel Hospital, Jos, in January 1970 when 28 cases occurred; five were hospital staff, and resulted in 14 deaths. Adding to the shock of these events was the fact that one of the fatal cases was Dr Jeanette Troup who had received and treated the original case from Lassa the previous year. The personal impact of these events has been covered by J. G. Fuller.[61]

Between the first incident in January 1969 and the end of July 1978 there have been 17 reported episodes involving 386 cases and 105 deaths,[166] giving an overall case-fatality rate of 27.2 per cent. Major studies have thrown light on the epidemiology of the disease which has proved to be a zoonosis, probably transmitted to man from a rodent reservoir which may be the rat *Mastomys natalensis*, widely distributed throughout Africa. The disease is endemic in certain areas of West Africa, particularly Sierra Leone, Liberia and the Jos plateau of Nigeria, while other areas of Nigeria together with Guinea, Senegal, Mali, Central African Empire and Zaire have been implicated on historical or serological evidence.[79] An isolation has also been made from *M. natalensis* in Mozambique.[98]

The mode of spread of infection among rodents has not been elucidated but the virus has been shown to establish a long-term viruria which, in conjunction with the scavenging habits of rats, could well provide the basic mechanism. The same mechanism may also be operated in rodent-to-man transfer of infection since the majority of native houses and dwelling compounds are heavily infested with rats. Here, the portal of entry might be either the gastrointestinal tract from contaminated food or water, or the respiratory tract from the inhalation of aerosols derived from dried infected urine.[79]

Clinically, the disease has an undramatic and uncharacteristic onset with fever, headache and muscle pains. The more characteristic signs do not appear until after the sixth day of persistent fever which has failed to respond to antibiotic treatment. At this time, a severe pharyngitis develops with ulceration of the buccal and pharyngeal mucosae, deepening prostration and dehydration, nausea, vomiting and diarrhoea. In severe cases, there may be a rash with petechial haemorrhages and the development of a general haemorrhagic tendency. The blood picture shows an early leukopaenia and thrombocytopaenia but the white count tends to rise above normal levels as the disease progresses.[58, 74, 76, 78]

Viraemia is present throughout the clinical illness and may approach 10^4 TCD50/ml.[65, 74, 76, 79] Virus is also present in the pharyngeal secretions and in serous effusions which may occur during the course of the illness. Viruria occurs in most patients and, in recovered cases, may persist for many weeks.[71, 78, 79]

Person-to-person transfer of infection has most commonly occurred as a result of close nursing and clinical contact which probably involves blood, body fluids or pharyngeal secretions. In view of the presence of virus in the pharynx and the occurrence of demonstrable pneumonitis, respiratory transmission is also a possibility, but severe lung involvement seems to be unusual and, in practice, respiratory transmission appears to be rare.

With the recognition of the endemic status of the disease and the occurrence of many non-fatal and even subclinical infections, the apparent case-fatality rate has been progressively revised downwards towards a hospital case-fatality rate of about 25 per cent and an infection-fatality rate of less than 5 per cent.[60, 70, 72]

Of the 17 recorded episodes (see Table 3), 11 were hospital outbreaks involving a total of 57 cases with 25 deaths (43.8 per cent). Two were laboratory infections, two were individual community-acquired infections with no secondary transmission and two were prolonged community outbreaks studied over periods of two years and three years respectively.[60, 70] A number of hospital infections also occurred during these last two studies but were secondary to the ongoing community outbreaks. The observed case-fatality rate of 43.8 per cent among nosocomial (hospital acquired) infections is in sharp contrast to the rate of 24.3 per cent in community-acquired infections.

Since February 1969, eight cases have been flown to Europe or the US. One of these was a 'dedicated' air evacuation to Frankfurt, West Germany, but the other seven travelled by scheduled commercial flights. Five of these cases were infectious when they travelled and only one was segregated from the other passengers at any stage of the journey. The exception was the third case of the original series who was gravely ill at the time and occupied the first-class cabin as a stretcher case separated only by a curtain from the other passengers. She was accompanied by a nurse and a physician, Dr Lyle Conrad of CDC, Atlanta.

There was no transmission of infection. Over 1,200 of the contacts of the other four infectious cases were traced and placed under surveillance; again there was no transmission of infection.[166]

The facts presented can leave no doubt that Lassa fever is an extremely dangerous disease with an apparently high potential for nosocomial spread, especially to hospital staff caring for infected patients. Outside the hospital, spread of infection to contacts seems to be much more limited. The pattern suggests that the degree of hazard which the disease represents to countries outside the endemic areas can best be assessed by considering separately the nosocomial and community aspects since there is a fundamental difference in the epidemiology of the disease in these two situations, the nosocomial results from person-to-person transmission while the community is predominantly a rodent-based zoonosis.

Each of the episodes will be examined to determine what light it sheds on these two aspects of the hazard, particularly to the mode of transmission in each case and to the transmission rate in relation to the numbers at risk. This last factor has been largely overlooked but is clearly of critical importance in determining the epidemic potential of the disease. In most reports it has tended to become submerged in detailed consideration of instances of transmission to the exclusion of instances of failure of transmission where this might have been expected to occur. The resulting concentration on the positive instances has tended to create an impression of high infectivity out of proportion to the true situation. This is especially the case in the early reports which coloured the first impressions of the disease. The episodes under discussion are listed in Table 3, modified from Monath[79] and Galbraith.[166]

Individual episodes

Episode 1[58]

Case 1 was a missionary nurse who became ill at Lassa on 12 January 1969. The mode of infection was not determined but was probably nosocomial. The patient developed a severe pharyngitis on 20 January and was nursed in her room until she was flown to Jos on 25 January. She died the next day. Until 20 January this nurse continued with her normal duties despite her increasing illness and, on 19 January, carried out a delivery in the maternity unit. At this time she must have had a high concentration of virus in her throat. From 20 to 25 January she was cared for by the mission doctor and staff under extremely basic conditions without protective clothing of any kind and, indeed, her colleagues were unaware of the infectious nature of the disease. There were no further cases at the hospital.

Table 3 Lassa fever episodes

Episode	Date	Place	Type and mode of infection (Index case)	Secondary cases	Tertiary cases	Deaths/ Cases	Contacts not infected	References
1	February 1969	Lassa, Jos	Nosocomial?	1 nurse – finger abrasion	1 nurse – autopsy and nursing	2/3	Not recorded	58
2	June 1969	New Haven	Laboratory infection	0	0	0/1	Not recorded (laboratory, hospital and family)	71
3	November 1969	New Haven	Laboratory infection	0	0	1/1	Not recorded (family and hospital)	61
4	January to February 1970	Jos	Community acquired	23 patients – visitors 18 Hospital staff (including one autopsy accident)	5 All close relatives and household contacts	13/28 (46%)	26 hospital staff 140 community	51, 91
5	October 1970 to October 1972	Panguma (Tongo)	Study of endemic community infection and hospitals. Transmission: Community Rodent-to-man Nosocomial Close contact	10 Nosocomial: visitors 5 in-patients 1 out-patients 4 Serologically positive: Panguma: 6/24 nurses 1/3 technicians 5/27 other staff Serabu 4/31 Nixon 4/64 Govt. Hospital 0/26 Eastern Clinic 0/19	None recorded	24/63 (38%)	194/214	60
6	1972	Panguma (London)	Nosocomial – pricked finger with needle after taking blood from moribund patient	0	0	0/1	Not recorded. Hospital and commercial flight but probably not infectious	96

Table 3 – *continued*

Episode	Date	Place	Type and mode of infection (Index case)	Secondary cases	Tertiary cases	Deaths/Cases	Contacts not infected	References
7	June 1971	Serabu (Liverpool)	Nosocomial – no details	0	0	0/1	Many hospital staff and visitors. Commercial flight when convalescent	62
8	September 1971	Seghwema (Burton, Lincs)	Nosocomial – physician no details	0	0	0/1	Numbers not recorded. Commercial flight on 4th day while very ill. Hospital in Lincs, UK	62
9	March April 1973	Zorzor Liberia	Community acquired	10 Patients 3 Hospital staff 7 All close contacts with gross contamination.	None definite but?2 infants of Lassa cases; both died.	4/11 (36%)	123/129 patients 14/21 staff	74, 75
10	January 1974	Onitsha Nigeria	Community acquired – student	1 Physician caring for index case	1 Physician. Performed tracheostomy on secondary case	1/3	Not recorded. Dedicated air-evacuation to Frankfurt	49, 88
11	January 1975	Vom Nigeria	Nosocomial. 3 cases	0	0	1/3	Not recorded	92
12	January 1975	Zonkwa Nigeria	Nosocomial. Physician flew to UK by commercial flight. Died after arrival	0	0	1/1	361	Woodruff quoted in 79

Table 3 – *continued*

Episode	Date	Place	Type and mode of infection (Index case)	Secondary cases	Tertiary cases	Deaths/ Cases	Contacts not infected	References
13	January 1973 to March 1976	Panguma Segbwema Sierra Leone	Study of endemic community infection and hospitals. Rodent-to-man transmission Nosocomial – close contact	Nosocomial only Serology: Panguma: 13/50 close 0/25 slight 0/5 techs Serabu: 2/95 staff Nixon: 4/64 staff	None recorded	55/ 264 (21%)	216/234 staff	70
14	January 1976	Sierra Leone	Community acquired. Peace Corps worker. Commercial flight to US via London. 553 contacts. Urine positive after arrival. Very ill during flight from Africa to London	0	0	0/1	552	100, 56
15	June 1976	Nigeria (London)	Community acquired. Engineer. Not seriously ill. Adm. to general hospital in London UK. Urine found positive	0	0	0/1	300	174
16	November 1977	Zaria Nigeria	Nosocomial. Physician	0	0	0/1	Not recorded	Bowen quoted in 166

Case 2 was a staff nurse at the Bingham Hospital, Jos, who cared for case 1 during the night after her arrival in Jos. During this time she swabbed out the patient's throat using a swab wrapped around her index finger, which she had pricked earlier that day. It is very likely that this was the route by which she became infected. She became ill after an eight-day incubation period and died on the eleventh day of her illness. During her illness she must have had a number of close contacts with the nursing and medical staff of the hospital and visitors. Of these unrecorded contacts only one of the nurses caring for her developed the infection.

Case 3 was the head nurse of the hospital. She had assisted at the autopsy of case 1 and nursed case 2. She became ill seven days after the death of case 2 and was presumably infected from that case rather than from the autopsy. Her contacts are not recorded from the onset of her illness on 20 February until she was flown to New York on 3 March, but there must have been many. No one became infected.

The flight was on a Pan-American Boeing 707 where the patient occupied the first-class cabin with a nurse from Jos and a doctor. She was critically ill at the time and must have been 'highly infectious' in terms of the presence of virus in her pharynx. The passengers in the economy-class cabin did not come face-to-face with the patient although they were only separated from her by a curtain, and would therefore be classified as 'remote' contacts. After perfunctory formalities at the airport the patient was taken to the Presbyterian Hospital in New York where she was cared for under standard conditions of 'full isolation', the staff and the one permitted visitor, her sister, wore 'full' protective clothing including cap, gown, gloves and mask. These procedures represented the normal standard isolation precautions recommended by the American Hospital Association[177] and fall considerably short of those later adopted by the Hospital for Tropical Diseases in London and those now recommended. As part of the clinical management of the case a wide range of laboratory examinations were carried out in the hospital's diagnostic laboratories by standard techniques. No transmission of infection occurred in either the aircraft or the hospital. These three cases are fully reported by Frame *et al.*[58]

Episode 2[71]

Specimens from the cases of the first episode reached the Yale Arbovirus Research Unit at Yale University, New Haven, Connecticut, on 9 March and were inoculated to suckling and adult mice and tissue culture. Dr Jordi Casals took personal charge of the animal work and carried out the isolation attempts in mice. He fell ill on 9 June and became steadily worse until he was admitted to the Presbyterian Hospital on 15 June. He was placed in 'full' isolation similar to that used for case 3. During the course of his very severe illness Dr Casals underwent a wide range of laboratory investigations and clinical monitoring procedures. On 18 June he received a plasma transfusion from case 3. His clinical condition improved and he was discharged from hospital 30 days after admission. Prior to his final discharge, however, he left the hospital to stay with his family for a few days, but was readmitted when it was found that a urine specimen taken on day 32 still contained virus.

Although the precise route of infection in this case must remain a matter of speculation there were clearly ample opportunities for laboratory-acquired infection in the animal handling techniques used. It must be remembered that the work was being carried out before there was a full awareness of the dangers involved and the somewhat casual techniques used in the far less dangerous arbovirus work were utilized – for instance, spinning infected mice by the tail on the open bench without using gloves let alone a mask. It would even appear that infective virus-containing fluids were pipetted by mouth. Under these conditions the unwitting ingestion or inhalation of infective material, especially dust derived from dried infective mouse urine during animal handling, is almost inevitable. Any agent whose minimal infected dose is small, for instance, psittacosis virus, the rickettsiae, the brucellae or the glanders bacillus *Pfeifferella whitmori*, rapidly gain a special reputation for danger in the laboratory. Those like *Salmonella typhi* whose minimal infective dose is large can be handled with relative safety. The infection of Dr Casals and the nosocomial transmission to nurses caring for infected patients suggest that the minimal infective dose (MID) for Lassa virus is small but it still required almost three months of intensive work under hazardous conditions before this laboratory infection occurred. There was no transmission to any of Dr Casals' contacts either within the laboratory or outside it.

Episode 3[61]

Five months after Dr Casals' laboratory infection a second case occurred in the arbovirus unit. This time, a male technician, was not involved in the Lassa virus work although his wife was a trainee in the tissue culture laboratory where such work was being carried out. The mode of infection was never elucidated. Onset of illness in this patient was on the day before the laboratory closed for Thanksgiving when he and his wife travelled to his home in York, Pennsylvania. He became progressively worse over the holiday and during the following week, but did not appear to be critically ill and was nursed at home as a case of influenza. Even after admission to hospital the nature of his illness was not suspected so no special precautions were taken. It was not, in fact, until after his death on about the twelfth day of his illness that the diagnosis of Lassa fever was made by virus isolation.

There is no record of this patient's contacts but it is clear that he must have had intimate contact with his wife and close contact with other members of his family as well as numerous hospital contacts of varying degrees of closeness. The numbers involved are not stated but there was no transmission.

Discussion of Episodes 1–3. The five cases comprising this initial series of infections deserve special consideration because they engendered the extreme alarm, started by the press, which now surrounds this disease. Examining the events associated with the first three cases shows clearly that the risk of infection was related to close nursing contact, but when the numbers of such contacts are considered, the transmission rate was clearly low. This pattern suggests that transmission was not by the respiratory route. The type of mechanism likely to be involved is suggested by the second case.

Severe pharyngeal inflammation with much pain and copious secretions would require frequent nursing care. If high virus concentrations are present in the pharynx and mouth, this could be very dangerous with a virus capable of infecting by direct access through skin abrasions or via contaminated fingers to the nose, mouth or conjunctiva. It is likely that any of these portals of entry could lead to infection with Lassa virus. The fact that no transmission occurred during the commercial flight of the second case also strongly suggests that this patient was not infective by the respiratory route.

The precise mechanisms of infection in the two laboratory episodes can only be guessed at but are not altogether beyond speculation considering the lack of special precautions. More surprising than their occurrence is the length of time which elapsed before they did so and their failure to transmit infection to any of the numerous close and even intimate contacts with whom they must have associated.

Episode 4[51, 91]

The next appearance of the disease was a hospital outbreak at the Evangel Hospital, Jos, Nigeria. The Evangel is a 56-bed hospital built in the shape of a letter 'T'. The left arm, Ward A, was the site of the outbreak. Ward A and the right arm, Ward B, were open wards while the upright wing contained a series of four double rooms. There was also a separate private pavilion.

In January 1970 a patient was admitted to Ward A diagnosed as having pneumonia with severe and extensive lung involvement. This patient was identified by retrospective analysis as being the probable index case of Lassa fever and when she was eventually traced she was found to have Lassa antibodies. The subsequent case incidence suggests that this woman infected 16 patients and staff who in turn passed the infection to another 5. One out-patient also appeared to have been infected. A twenty-third case, Dr Jeanette Troup, was the result of an autopsy accident which caused the direct inoculation of virus through a knife wound. Five further cases occurred outside the hospital in intimate home contacts of patients on Ward A.

Discussion of Episode 4. The *Index case* in this episode was of community acquired infection from an unknown source. The endemic situation in Nigeria has not as yet been investigated.

Secondary cases. The occurrence of secondary infections in 5 members of staff and 16 patients in the one ward suggests at first sight direct contact transmission to nursing staff with indirect transmission by them to the other patients – a pattern which would follow the classical mechanism of transmission of staphylococcal infection in surgical wards. Three facts, however, run counter to this explanation:

(1) The nursing staff affected did not have the same intimate degree of contact with the index case as did the two nurses who had become infected in the same hospital in the previous year during the first Lassa episode.

(2) The same nursing staff looked after the patients on all three wards.

(3) The bedpans and other utensils were also shared between all three wards.

Since the cases were restricted to Ward A it seems that contact transmission through faulty nursing procedures was unlikely to have been the mechanism of spread. The possibility of a common source outbreak through contaminated food could also be eliminated since, in common with the practice in most similar hospitals, food was the responsibility of relatives and was not supplied by the hospital.

Although the mode of transmission could not be identified with certainty on epidemiological grounds, it was considered that in this instance there was a real possibility of respiratory transmission. The index case had been admitted as a case of pneumonia with extensive lung involvement and a persistent cough which could have generated a highly infective aerosol. Moreover, the patient was so positioned in the ward that air movement would have drawn such an aerosol across other patients and into the body of the ward.

This episode is most important since it stands alone in suggesting a real likelihood of respiratory infection in person-to-person transmission. If this did in fact occur, it seems certain that it was due to the response of the index case to infection, in that the patient developed an exceptionally severe pneumonic involvement, rather than to a change in the characteristics of the virus itself. Had it been due to the development of pneumotropism by the virus it is unlikely that the outbreak would have burned itself out at the stage of the few tertiary cases which occurred in community contacts.

Episode 5[60]

This was the continued outbreak on the Tongo area of Sierra Leone which was investigated by Fraser *et al.*[60] and is discussed on pages 83–85.

Episode 6[96]

A missionary nurse at the Panguma Catholic hospital pricked her finger with a hypodermic needle which she had just used to take blood from a patient with a high fever. The patient died the next day. There had already been at least eight deaths in similarly ill patients during the previous six months. The nurse was cared for without isolation since such facilities were not available at the Panguma hospital. On day 28 of her illness, when she was still clinically very unwell but probably not infectious, she travelled to London by commercial aircraft. There was no transmission of infection to any person at the hospital or on the flight. The mode of infection in this case is clear and the incident is one of several which demonstrate the ability of the virus to infect by direct inoculation into the tissues.

Episode 7[62]

In June 1971, a nurse at the Serabu Hospital, Sierra Leone, acquired Lassa fever. She was treated without isolation or precautions in a convent where she had numerous visitors. No sickness or antibodies were detected retrospectively among her known contacts, although actual numbers are not stated. She was transferred to England on a commercial flight on day 28 of her illness when she was probably no longer infectious. There was no transmission.

Episode 8[62]

In September 1971, a missionary physician at the Serabu Hospital contracted Lassa fever and travelled to London by commercial flight on the fourth day of his illness when he was feeling extremely ill and was in the acute stage of the disease. When he arrived in England he was admitted to a small hospital in Lincolnshire where he was treated without special precautions and given 'normal care' for a virus infection. He was discharged after 10 days. Contacts aboard the aircraft were not traced since the nature of his illness was not known at that time and no further cases occurred.

In both of the last two episodes infection was nosocomial but no specific incident would be identified to account for them.

Episode 9[74, 75]

This episode was a striking nosocomial outbreak with 11 cases, seven among hospital staff, and four deaths. The index case was a pregnant woman admitted with fever, vomiting, abdominal pain and vaginal bleeding. She was admitted to the maternity ward which she shared with other patients admitted for delivery or for complications of pregnancy. The index case aborted before delivery and underwent dilatation and curettage (D&C). This event was followed by the occurrence of Lassa fever in seven members of the hospital staff and three other patients on the obstetrical ward. All the staff members involved had had heavy exposure by the changing of maternity pads and general hygienic duties, including handling and measuring urine. Nursing technique was not of a high order and the CDC Report[84] carries the following statement:

> One of the fatal cases was in an American missionary nurse. She had performed the D&C on the index case and had gotten blood and lochia on open varicose ulcers on her legs.

Discussion of Episode 9. Although Monath *et al.*[75] state that 'the mode of spread was not defined' there can be little doubt in view of experience in hospital infection control that gross environmental contamination of ward and patients must have occurred by way of the hands of the attendant staff. This conclusion is supported by the pattern of spread of infection determined serologically among contacts inside and outside the hospital. Among 21 members of the hospital staff, four had 'heavy' exposure and three had 'moderate' exposure; all seven became infected. Twelve had 'slight' exposure and two had 'none' – none of them became infected.

Outside the hospital it was found that 6 of 129 people who had contact with the maternity ward were serologically positive although none had suffered clinical illness.

There were no tertiary cases and no cases in other wards of the hospital. Infection was thus confined to the one ward and its contacts, and clinical illness to those in the heavily contaminated area. There was no evidence of respiratory spread of infection and no spread beyond the immediate ward contacts.

Episode 10[49, 88]

In January 1974, a 19-year-old student in Onitsha, Nigeria, contracted Lassa fever by community infection whose nature could not be determined. The physician who cared for him at the Onitsha hospital became infected and died, and a second physician who performed a tracheostomy on the moribund second case also became infected but survived.

Among the staffs of five hospitals in the area, 258 persons were serologically tested including 92 who had a high degree of contact with the infected patients, 81 with a low degree of contact, and 66 with no contact as well as 9 community contacts and 10 others with no contact. None were found to possess antibodies.

Discussion of Episode 10. The mechanism of infection of the index case was not identified nor was that of the first physician, although the latter was clearly nosocomial. The second physician, however, performed a tracheostomy on his colleague and this in the extremity of an illness with gross pharyngitis and laryngeal obstruction would almost certainly have given rise to an intense aerosol of infected blood and tracheal secretions. Infection might, therefore, have been either respiratory or from contact with infected blood. Again, the absence of transmission to any of the large number of close contacts is noteworthy.

Episode 11[92]

In January 1975, three nosocomial infections occurred in Vom, Nigeria. The mechanism of infection was not determined. There was no spread of infection to contacts of these three cases.

Episode 12[79]

In January 1975, an English missionary physician contracted infection in Zonkwa, Nigeria, and was flown to London by commercial flight at the height of his illness. After arrival in

England he was admitted to the Hospital for Tropical Diseases in London where he died. The 361 contacts, mostly passengers on his flight, were traced and placed under surveillance. No transmission occurred.

Episode 13 (see page 85)

Episode 14[100, 56]

In February 1976, a female American Peace Corps worker in Sierra Leone contracted Lassa fever. At the time she was living with her husband in quarters where a previous case had occurred the year before.

While she was still sick, on day 19 of her illness, she and her husband travelled to Washington, D.C. via Heathrow, London, where they had a four-hour stopover. After spending the weekend with her husband in a Washington hotel she was admitted to the George Washington University Hospital where she was placed in strict isolation.

Apart from her husband, who accompanied her until she was admitted to hospital, 552 contacts were traced. All were placed under surveillance. Of these contacts, 30 were in Freetown, Sierra Leone; 115 were passengers and crew on the flight from Freetown to Heathrow; 233 were passengers and crew on the flight from London to Washington and 85 were in downtown Washington. There was no transmission of the disease. Twenty-one of the Washington contacts were considered to be at high risk and were serologically tested. None developed antibody.

Discussion of Episode 14. The mechanism of this community-acquired infection was not determined but in view of the following studies which have demonstrated the enzootic status of the disease in Sierra Leone it seems likely that infection was derived from the rodent reservoir, especially as a previous case had occurred in the same quarters. Whatever its origin there is little doubt that the patient was seriously ill during her entire journey from Africa to Washington and during her weekend in Washington. This probability is strengthened by the fact that Lassa virus was isolated from her urine on 3 March, day 23 of her illness, after her admission to hospital. The degree to which she was likely to have been shedding virus at the time of her journey is in some doubt despite the later demonstration but nevertheless she accumulated a formidable number of contacts, some of them close, during the course of her illness and travels. Yet she did not transmit the infection to a single person – not even to her husband who was an intimate contact throughout.

Episode 15[174]

In June 1976, an engineer flew to London from Nigeria by scheduled flight and was admitted to St Mary's Hospital with pyrexia of unknown origin. However, he remained in the hospital in an open ward until it was found that he was excreting Lassa virus in his urine. He was then transferred to a plastic isolator at London's Coppetts Wood Hospital and 300 contacts were traced and placed under surveillance. There was no transmission of infection. This case is one of the few mild cases of Lassa infection recorded in a white person. Although the patient was ambulatory during much of his illness, he did not transmit infection.

Episode 16[166]

A missionary physician at Zaria, Nigeria, contracted Lassa fever, presumably by nosocomial infection. No details are available.

Episodes 5 and 13[60, 70]

The episodes so far considered have been individual clear-cut events arising from identifiable index cases and have either been individual infection without transmission or have been self-limiting outbreaks with no transmission beyond the third generation. Although hospital transmission has been the basis of all but four of the episodes, they must nevertheless have reflected some unrecognized endemic situation in the community. In northern Nigeria this is still the state of affairs, but in Sierra Leone two groups of workers have carried out extensive community studies which have greatly elucidated the endemic disease pattern.

Episode 5[60]

The study by Fraser *et al.*[60] is based upon the hospital records in the Tongo-Panguma group of towns for the two-year period from 1 October 1970. The population of the area is about 14,500 and the people live in family groups of from 1 to 45 members in compounds of 1 to 4 buildings with 4 to 10 rooms per compound. The houses are, for the most part, mud and wattle constructions with cement floors and thatch or corrugated iron roofing. The life of the community revolves around the National Diamond Mining Company and the living standards are relatively high. Nevertheless, the area is heavily infested with rats which invade the living compounds and it was this study that incriminated *Mastomys natalensis* as a carrier, and possibly natural reservoir of the Lassa virus.

From hospital records 63 cases were identified which met the exacting criteria applied for identification of Lassa fever cases (see Table 4). Twenty-four of these cases died to give a case-fatality rate of 38 per cent. The series included nine pregnant women of whom six (67 per cent) died.

Field studies revealed that the cases were not grouped but had been scattered throughout the area and there were only three compounds where more than one case had occurred, each had two cases.

Table 4   Tongo-Panguma episodes
(distribution of cases by households)

Study	Total cases	Total households	Households with:				1 case only (in %)
			6 cases	3 cases	2 cases	1 case	
Fraser *et al.*	63	60	—	—	3	57	95
Keane and Gilles	134	123	1	1	4	117	95
Total	197	183	1	1	7	174	95

In 57 compounds single cases only occurred and 50 of the 63 cases gave no evidence of contact with previous cases of Lassa fever. Serological investigation, however, did reveal a degree of clustering of positive reactors in compounds where cases had occurred, and within the compounds there was a suggestion of clustering within the room where the index case had slept. There was heavy rodent infestation; rats frequently occupied the thatch and rafters, urinating and defaecating freely upon the family below, so it was not possible to determine whether the clustering was due to common exposure or to person-to-person spread.

In all, 6 per cent of 255 persons tested were found to be seropositive although only 0.2 per cent had suffered serious clinical illness.

Among the hospital-associated cases, one case had occurred in a patient hospitalized for delivery, four in patients attending out-patient clinics and five among visitors to the hospital wards. A serological survey of the hospital staff in the area gave the results shown in Table 5.[104] Of the six nurses at the Panguma hospital who had antibodies, four had had severe illnesses but none of the other seropositive persons had been hospitalized for febrile illness.

Episode 13 [70]

In the second study, carried out by Keane and Gilles,[70] covering the period from January 1973 to March 1976, 156 patients admitted to the Panguma Hospital were identified as probable cases of Lassa fever. In this series the case-fatality rate for men and non-pregnant women was 16.2 per cent, but the fatality rate for pregnant women was 50 per cent.

In tracing the background of these infections Keane and Gilles paid particular attention to the issue of transmission under varying circumstances with results which confirm and extend those of Fraser *et al.*[60]

Household transmission. The pattern of infection in households again illustrates the isolated and sporadic nature of the individual cases. Out of 134 cases whose homes could be traced, 117 were single cases from individual households and only six households had more than one case. Of these six, one household had six cases, one had three and four had two each (see Table 4, p. 84). The incidence of seropositivity in infected households was, however, twice that in the general community – 13 per cent as opposed to 6 per cent. Keane and Gilles concluded that the pattern suggested rodent-to-man transfer of infection rather than person-to-person spread.

Hospital transmission. In the hospital, Lassa fever cases presented in the overcrowded out-patient clinic and from there were admitted to the hospital wards. Sixty per cent of the Lassa cases were admitted directly to a four-bed isolation ward which was separated from the general ward only by a linen screen, while 40 per cent had to be barrier-nursed in the general wards where no isolation was possible. Relatives, who provided the food for the patients twice each day, and all visitors, gained access to the isolation ward through the general wards. Visitors and relatives never wore protective clothing and medical and nursing staff seldom did. During the three years of the study an average of 5.6 cases of Lassa fever were admitted each month, and only one month, November 1973, passed without at least one case being admitted.

TABLE 5   Serological survey of Tongo-Panguma hospitals
(Fraser *et al.* 1974[60])

Hospital	Staff tested	Number tested	Number positive	Per cent positive
Panguma	Nurses	24	6	25
	Laboratory technicians	3	1	—
	Others	27	5	18
	Sub-total	54	12	22
Serabu	All	31	4	13
Nixon Memorial	All	57	4	7
Government	All	26	0	—
Eastern Clinic	All	19	0	—
	Sub-total	133	8	6
Total		187	20	10.7

(Keane and Gilles, 1977[70])

Hospital	Staff tested	Number tested	Number positive	Per cent positive
Panguma	Close contacts	50	15 (2 deaths)	30
	Technicians	5	0	—
Serabu	Staff	98	2	2
Tongo	Staff	28	1	3.6

Patients. From the figures it is is evident that, during the period studied, over 3,000 patients were exposed to continuous risk of cross-infection from active cases of Lassa fever, many of which were fatal. In spite of this there were only two cases of hospital-acquired infection among them. These occurred when a patient in the general ward infected a woman in the next bed who then infected her baby who was breastfed. Also during this period a number of patients suspected of having Lassa fever, but later shown not to have the disease, were nursed in the isolation ward along with proven Lassa cases without acquiring infection.

Visitors. Serological studies in the Panguma area[60, 70] suggest that over 90 per cent of the population do not possess demonstrable antibodies against Lassa virus so it may be presumed that the majority of the visitors and relatives were susceptible to infection, yet here again only one possible case of infection was discovered.

Hospital staff. Among 75 members of the hospital staff, 50 were close contacts of Lassa patients and of these 15 became infected and two died. In Serabu and Tongo hospitals only 2 of 98 and 1 of 28 staff respectively were found to be seropositive by complement fixation testing.

Finally, in the laboratory, no special precautions were taken in the handling of specimens from Lassa patients yet none of the five technicians had antibodies against Lassa virus.

Discussion of Episodes 5 and 13. There are very clear similarities in the results of these two studies and despite the caution of both groups of workers in their interpretation of the mechanism of transmission of infection, from the point of view of this report certain conclusions can be drawn with confidence. First, it is evident that there are two epidemiologically distinct patterns to be considered, one in the community and the other in the hospital setting.

Community pattern. Both studies show a marked predominance of single cases of infection from individual households albeit with a clustering of seropositive persons in association with the index cases. There can be little doubt that the index cases themselves were of zoonotic origin from the rodent reservoir, but the cause of the serological clustering must remain in doubt. Whether it is caused by person-to-person transmission within the family or exposure to a common source of infection, the pattern is clearly that of self-limited episodes of a disease with very low transmissibility even in overcrowded populations living in primitive conditions of hygiene. Moreover, the findings in both studies that 94 per cent of the population who are seronegative suggest that the low transmissibility was not due to herd immunity in the population at risk, but is an intrinsic characteristic of the disease itself. It further suggests that the disease is not easily transmitted by the respiratory route and therefore its epidemic potential by direct person-to-person transmission is low. This conclusion in respect of a predominantly susceptible community subjected to an incidence of over 100 fresh index cases every year is of considerable importance in assessing the epidemic threat arising from sporadic introductions into communities outside the African continent.

Hospital pattern. In contrast to the rodent-to-man transmission of the community epidemiological pattern, hospital transmission must be predominantly person-to-person and again the two studies closely agree on incidence, although Fraser *et al.* discovered a slightly higher incidence of cross-infection among patients and visitors. With respect to hospital staff Fraser *et al.* found an overall incidence of seropositivity of 9 per cent against 10 per cent by Keane and Gilles, while the figures for close contacts, including nurses and laboratory technicians, were 25.9 per cent and 30 per cent respectively. These of course are cumulative figures and, if it be assumed that the staff remained constant and that all the infections occurred after the studies began, they would represent a maximum incidence of infection of only 10 per cent per year despite continued exposure under the far from ideal conditions described.

These findings suggest that the concept of Lassa fever as a disease of high infectivity to hospital and especially nursing personnel, is not well-founded.

Mortality. Both studies reported case-fatality rates lower than those previously observed. These were 38 per cent in the study by Fraser *et al.* and 20 per cent in that of Keane and Gilles. The former workers estimated that the infection-fatality rate was less than 5 per cent and the most recent findings of McCormick in Sierra Leone suggest a lower figure still.[72] Although still high, these figures are lower than those previously reported and are well below the yellow fever case-fatality rates observed in Nigeria in the epidemic of 1969–70.

2. Case-fatality rate

Estimates of the case-fatality rate based upon hospitalized cases of infection have declined steadily since the original episodes of 1969 when three out of the first five known cases died to give a fatality rate of 60 per cent (see Table 5). It now seems that the estimates even from the Sierra Leone studies[60, 70] may still be too high since McCormick and Johnson have reported[72] that about 50 per cent of all patients with feverish illness admitted to the Kenema study hospitals, Sierra Leone, were suffering from Lassa fever. This finding must still be fitted into the whole community picture, but the previous studies[60, 70] have already indicated from serological surveys that Lassa virus gives rise to a considerable incidence of minor illness and even subclinical infection and Fraser *et al.*[60] estimated that the infection-fatality rate, taking serological findings into account, was less than 5 per cent. McCormick and Johnson[72] reported a fatality rate of about 20 per cent in hospitalized cases but found that about 40 per cent of the adult population was seropositive.

One further observation of these studies requires special mention. It appears that pregnancy exerts a potentiating effect on the disease process. The numbers are small but suggest that the fatality rate in pregnant women is about double that in men and non-pregnant women.

3. Community incidence

The community incidence in the Panguma-Tongo region was studied by Fraser *et al.*[60] during the 1970–72 outbreak. They found a seropositivity rate of 6 per cent in a survey of 255 individuals from control compounds where no cases of Lassa fever had occurred as compared with 13 per cent among 206 individuals from case compounds. These figures were very similar to those found by Keane and Gilles,[70] and contrasted strongly with the estimated case incidence of 0.2 per cent and mortality rate of 0.08 per cent over the two-year period. Interpretation is, however, difficult since the findings relate to the first part of an epidemic curve starting in February 1970 and rising steadily until the end of 1972 when the study was concluded. It must be presumed that the incidence was considerably in excess of the interepidemic level, but the figures are important in showing the limited epidemic potential of the disease even among a susceptible rat-infested community.

4. Seasonal incidence

There is as yet insufficient information for an assessment of trends in seasonal incidence although there is a suggestion[70] that two peaks may occur, the first during January – March and the second in June – July.

5. Ecology

Information about the ecology of the disease is far from complete. The evidence so far suggests that the natural reservoir of the virus is the multimammate rat *Mastomys natalensis* which has been the only animal carrier identified among 26 species tested in Sierra Leone and Nigeria. The numbers of animals tested so far have, however, been small and their geographical area limited. The positive findings in the case of *Mastomys* itself have been conspicuously grouped in relation to infected compounds. In Tongo for instance, 10 of the 14 positive animals came from two infected households. While there can be no doubt that this species acts as a reservoir, some epidemiologists believe there is insufficient evidence to identify it positively as the primary reservoir for the virus. In the first place the grouping of positive animals could have resulted from transmission of the virus from human cases rather than through a rat-to-rat epizootic cycle and also the extensive distribution of *Mastomys* throughout the African continent does not accord well with the apparent localization of the disease in northwest Africa.

In practical terms, however, whatever may ultimately prove to be the primary reservoir of the virus it must be accepted that *Mastomys* function at least as a link reservoir, and that its close association with living compounds in the endemic areas, taken in association with the findings of the Panguma-Tongo studies,[60, 70] make it the most likely immediate source of infection for the great majority of the human cases in the community.

This positive conclusion should be considered together with the negative evidence suggesting that the other animal species commonly found in association with the human population in the endemic areas are virtually free from infection. This is despite the fact that the remainder of the 26 species tested, mostly rodents and bats, might be considered potential reservoirs, especially since occasional isolations have been made from the black rat, *Rattus rattus*, and the house mouse, *Mus. mirutoides*.[79] Clearly, the ecological threat which could result from the introduction of the virus into a virgin community such as North America would be closely bound up with the existence of susceptible species which might become infected and lead to the establishment of an enzootic state similar to that which followed the introduction of the plague bacillus into California.

6. Vector requirements

Arthropod vectors play a prominent part in transmitting infectious diseases in Africa, and *M. natalensis* which hagbours a number of ectoparasites of low host specificity, particularly *Xenopsylla philoxera*, is an important transmitter of plague in southern Africa. Under the conditions prevailing in most native compounds there would clearly be opportunity for free exchange of ectoparasites between rodents and man and it would be rash to dismiss the possibility of arthropod vector transmission even if it were a purely passive process similar to that of myxomatosis. Nevertheless, arthropods have not been incriminated in the transmission of Lassa fever and are clearly not a requirement in the disease cycle.

7. Mechanisms of transmission of infection

Transmission in the community. The mechanisms of transmission of infection either between rats or humans have not been precisely identified although a number of obvious possibilities exist. There are recent relevant experiences in the transmission of lymphocytic choriomeningitis reported from the US.[63] There have been three major outbreaks of this disease in laboratory and hospital personnel engaged in work on the passage of transmissible tumours in hamsters. In two of them the virus was initially derived not from the hamster stock itself but from the tumour tissue. The majority of the cases were in personnel concerned with handling the animals or their infected tissues, so they were liable to direct contamination with virus-containing materials. Others, however, were more remotely related to the work, which suggests that respiratory infection might have been involved. The most likely vehicle would then be a secondary aerosol derived from dried infectious urine or faeces and dispersed when handling the animals. Many rodents tend to urinate freely when disturbed or handled and *M. natalensis* is particularly noted for this type of behaviour.[67]

Arenaviruses are of low pathogenicity for their rodent hosts and tend to produce prolonged carrier states with persistent viruria which, through contamination of the food and general environment, would easily account for the transmission of virus through the rodent community. Rats living in the roofs and rafters of native living quarters must similarly produce heavy environmental contamination to which both the rodents themselves and the human inhabitants would be freely exposed. In addition, *Mastomys* is widely utilized as a food item in Africa and catching and killing the animals is therefore associated with heavy urinary contamination.

This type of contamination and its consequences are very well known to workers handling laboratory animals and are well illustrated by the reputation psittacosis virus has as a laboratory hazard. In this case virus is heavily shed in the diarrhoeal faeces which contaminated the feathers and give rise to massive secondary aerosols when the birds are caught and handled. The same mechanism would almost certainly account for the laboratory infection of Dr Casals with Lassa virus.

Of critical importance is the question of person-to-person transmission since this is the key factor in the epidemic hazard to the human community. Community infection in the endemic areas is dominated by the pattern of rodent-to-man transmission. However, Fraser *et al.* suggested that the clustering of seropositives among people who shared the sleeping accommodation of cases might be due to person-to-person transmission, possibly by the respiratory route. This possibility can neither be proved nor disproved on epidemiological grounds but, if it does occur it is infrequent and of little importance in the natural history of the observed community disease pattern. In the hospital situation, however, the reverse is true. Here rodent-to-man transmission may be discounted and only the possible mechanisms of person-to-person spread need to be considered.

Transmission in hospital. It will be clear from the analysis of individual episodes that there have been three principal types of transmission in the hospital context. The *first* has been direct inoculation of the virus through the skin as a result of accidental trauma. In most cases this has been due to the classical type of syringe-needle accident and in one instance to an autopsy accident. The second case of the first episode was probably infected through a pre-existing finger prick when the second patient used her ungloved hand to clear secretions from the first patient's ulcerated pharynx. This route of infection by direct trauma is obviously similar to that of Hepatitis B in the hospital setting and reflects the ubiquitous distribution of the virus throughout the body with high concentrations in the blood and tissue fluids.

Sore throat is a constant feature of onset and suggests that virus is regularly present in the pharynx early in the disease although its irregular isolation may imply that its concentration remains low until about the sixth day when gross inflammation and ulceration occur. Serous effusions contain virus and all blood-stained excretions or other materials contaminated by internal or external haemorrhage are highly infectious. Viruria is an inconstant feature but, when it occurs, it may persist for many weeks.

As a direct consequence of the active nursing care required, the vomiting and haemorrhagic diathesis and the high infectivity of the blood, the *second* frequent mode of nosocomial transmission has been as a result of close patient contact without evidence of specific trauma. The most conspicuous example of this was the outbreak at Zorzor in a maternity ward where the nursing techniques permitted gross contamination with infected blood, urine and lochia from Lassa-infected patients.

The precise portal of entry involved in infection by such close contact cannot be identified, but manual contamination of mouth or nose is a clear possibility. The presence of unrecorded or unnoticed skin abrasions is also a possibility as is the inhalation of aerosols produced by careless handling of contaminated materials or fomites.

The *third* type of transmission, airborne transmission through the agency of droplet nuclei derived from the respiratory tract of the patient, has not been proven to occur in Lassa fever but must be accepted as a real possibility in view of the Jos outbreak of February 1970. Clinical pneumonia and cough have not been reported as conspicuous features of the disease although microscopically evident pneumonitis appears to be frequently present and cough is an almost constant clinical feature. The suspect index case in the Jos outbreak was exceptional because the patient was admitted as a case of pneumonia with extensive lung involvement. In their report Carey *et al.*[51] were understandably cautious in their interpretation of the epidemiological data but their suggestion that the subsequent spread through the ward may have been due to airborne transmission must be seriously considered because of its implications for uncontrolled person-to-person spread. These implications will be further discussed in relation to containment.

8. *Infectious period of the patient*

Although precise virological information is still far from complete, it would appear from the clinical course that a generalized infection is present from the start of the illness and virus has been isolated from the blood as early as the second day.[76] At this time virus multiplication is probably occurring in the internal organs – probably the liver, spleen and bone marrow – even before internal mucosal surfaces such as those of the pharynx and gut become seriously involved.

Some degree of sore throat is present from the start but pharyngitis does not become severe until about the sixth day when gross inflammation and ulceration commence with whitish patches of exudate developing on the mucosa. Since internal generalization of the virus would not lead to external shedding and the faeces would not become infective until intestinal bleeding occurred, it is likely that the earliest dissemination of infectious virus would, in fact, be from the pharynx. How soon this would occur has not been determined, but virus has been isolated from throat swabs as early as the third and fourth days after onset.[65, 76] The virus concentration in throat swabs has been low compared with that in the serum. The clinical course suggests that virus shedding would tend to be slight during the early stages but would rise to a maximum when ulceration of the throat occurred after the sixth day. This suggestion is supported by the irregularity with which virus could be isolated from the throat.[78]

If this interpretation is correct, it implies that infectivity would be low during the early stages of the disease and would reach a maximum during the second week. This reasoning would also apply to the danger associated with coughing. Vomiting too increases in frequency and severity during the second week and the viral contamination of the vomit would increase with the rise in concentration of pharyngeal virus and the increasing haemorrhagic tendency. Finally, the urine may also become infective in the later stages. Both urine and pharynx may continue to harbour virus after the viraemia has cleared;[76, 79] the urinary carriage may continue for several weeks.[71, 76, 79, 100]

These somewhat disjointed and incomplete data must be interpreted with the understanding that infectivity is a complex phenomenon which depends on more than the demonstrable presence of virus in a particular location in the patient's body. For instance, viraemia is not in itself an infective threat; it becomes so only if blood escapes from the body as a result of haemorrhage or medical or surgical interference and it becomes an epidemic threat only if appropriate arthropod vectors are present. In Lassa fever the actual virological findings must be assessed in the light of other factors and it is then apparent that every case of transmission which can be positively identified has occurred from contact – usually very close contact – at the time of severe clinical disease. There is no instance of transmission during the first week of disease in spite of the fact that virus seems to be constantly present in the pharynx at this time, nor has there been a single identifiable instance of transmission due to carriage of virus in the urine. Without the slightest doubt the period of greatest danger is during the severe clinical illness from about the sixth day onwards and is related to close bodily contact with infective body fluids.

This conclusion has an important bearing on the question of transmissibility and therefore on public health response and patient management.

9. *Transmissibility*

Lassa fever is a zoonosis so its incidence in man reflects its enzootic or epizootic state in an animal reservoir or vector; in Lassa fever the reservoir is the rodent *Mastomys natalensis.* Transmissibility must, therefore, be considered at three levels: rodent-to-rodent, rodent and man and person-to-person within the human population.

Transmissibility between rodents. Evidence regarding the transmissibility of Lassa virus infection within the rodent population is almost completely lacking. Possible mechanisms have already been discussed and are not difficult to envisage but their impact can be judged only from the results of two field surveys of very limited scope. In the first survey, reported by Monath *et al.*[76] in relation to the Tongo-Panguma outbreak investigated by Fraser *et al.*,[60] 14 of 82 *Mastomys* were found to be infected but their local distribution was very uneven. In Panguma only 1 of 46 rats of this species was positive, while 13 of 35 were positive in Tongo. In Panguma, only six of the animals tested were captured in human habitations whereas in Tongo the figure was 39 of which 12, yielding 10 of the positives, were from two households which had had cases of the disease. It is not stated whether the other three isolates were also from infected households. In terms of rodent incidence these figures are uninterpretable and give no indication of transmissibility within the rodent species since the 10 positive rats from infected households could well have been infected from human rather than rodent sources. They indicate no more, in fact, than the susceptibility of *Mastomys* to infection by the virus.

The second survey was carried out by Wulff *et al.*[97] in Nigeria during November–December 1972 and March–April 1973, at which times no human cases of Lassa fever were recorded. Five of 20 *M. natalensis* from one location were found to be infected. Johnson suggests that the finding of virus in 2 of 10 *R. rattus* and 1 of 2 *Mus. minutoides* being positive, may have been due to error in species identification. These isolates confirm the zoonotic nature of the disease but are again too scanty to give any measure of prevalence from which conclusions regarding transmissibility within the rodent population could be drawn.

Transmissibility between rodent and man. The possible mechanisms of transmission of Lassa virus between *M. natalensis* and man ensure that transfer of infection is strongly dependent upon local conditions. Under the type of conditions prevailing in the Tongo-Panguma area where infestation in human living quarters is heavy, food hygiene is sketchy and food stores are unprotected against rodent invasion, there are many opportunities for transmission and the enzootic incidence will tend to be closely mirrored in the incidence of human cases.

In rural communities where for much of the year the rodent tends to inhabit fields, infection will be less frequent and probably more subject to seasonal variations relating to the harvest, hunting of *Mastomys* for food and its seasonal migration into houses when the fields are stripped of grain. In major cities where *Mastomys* tends to be evicted by *R. rattus*, human infection will be unusual.

These relatively simple patterns of transmission do not appear to be complicated in the case of Lassa fever by any potentiation resulting from arthropod vectors.

The implications of this rodent-man association for communities outside the African continent cannot be foreseen at this time. *Mastomys* is not native to North America or to Europe and there is no indication that it could become established in either continent if introduced. There is no knowledge about whether other wild rodent species indigenous to these areas could become infected and serve as reservoirs of the virus. Even if this could and did happen it seems likely that the general pattern of relatively distant human association with rodents would lead only to the sporadic type of zoonotic incidence now seen with tuleraemia and plague.

Person-to-person transmissibility. The most critical aspect of transmissibility is that of person-to-person spread since this determines the degree of epidemic risk which follows the introduction of Lassa fever into susceptible Western communities and also the nosocomial risk from hospitalized patients.

From the evidence already reviewed, it can now be accepted that the risk of person-to-person spread in the community as a whole is minimal. All the available evidence shows that person-to-person transmission even under the somewhat primitive and overcrowded conditions prevailing in the African communities investigated, is a very minor aspect of the epidemic picture if indeed it occurs at all. Even in the Zorzor incident, where there is a strong presumption of airborne spread among hospital patients and personnel, transmission outside the hospital was limited to very close contacts within the family setting. This is especially important; it shows that the nosocomial transmission must have been caused by special environmental circumstances and not to a mutational change conferring pneumotropism or enhanced respiratory transmissibility on the virus itself.

In the hospital the situation is different. Apart from the special circumstances of the Zorzor episode, person-to-person transmission to close contacts, especially nursing contacts, is a real hazard carrying a very grave risk. Even here, however, transmissibility is low and appears to be limited to very close contacts of a patient at the height of illness. Blood and body fluids are the vehicles through which the virus is spread and there is clearly a close parallel with the transmission of Hepatitis B in the hospital setting.

The analysis of episodes not only underlines the requirement for close contact, but also shows that not a single known case of transmission from an infectious patient, either in hospital or in the community, has occurred outside the African continent. Without exception the episodes of transmission have been under relatively primitive conditions where isolation procedures have not been applied, and the episodes are, in fact, more remarkable for the numbers of contacts who have not been infected than for the number who have contracted the disease. This is particularly striking in those instances where commercial flights of sick patients have generated contacts of every degree of closeness from the accompanying marriage partner and attendant medical staff to remote airport contacts.

The evidence leaves no doubt that the disease in its present form is incapable of sustained spread through even a fully susceptible population living under primitive conditions and so the threat of an uncontrollable epidemic resulting from the chance introduction of Lassa fever into a Western community may be safely discounted.

Biology

The causative agent

Identity

The virus of Lassa fever is an arenavirus. This group of viruses contains 10 known members, all of them animal pathogens. Of the 10, 4 are also capable of infecting man: LCM virus, causing lymphocytic choriomeningitis; Junin virus, causing Argentinian haemorrhagic fever; Machupo virus, causing Bolivian haemorrhagic fever; and Lassa virus, causing Lassa fever.

The group is defined by Murphy:[80]

> The viruses contain single-stranded RNA in four large pieces (and several smaller pieces) with a total molecular weight of approximately 3.6×10^6. The viruses have four major polypeptides (two of which are glucosylated) and contain lipid and carbohydrates. The virion density is 1.17–1.18 g/ml in sucrose and the virion sedimentation coefficients are 325–500S. Infectivity is labile to lipid solvents, acids (pH 5.5) and radiation (ultra-violet and gamma). The virions have a unique morphology in thin section; they are spherical or pleomorphic and range in diameter from 50 to 300 nm (mean 110–130 nm). The particles have a unit-membrane envelope covered with club-shaped projections 10 nm in length and have a varying number of electron dense granules within an otherwise unstructured interior. These granules, 20–25 nm in diameter, have been shown to be ribosomes. Viral constituents synthesis takes place in the cytoplasm, often with inclusion body formation; maturation occurs via budding, primarily from plasma membranes. The viruses of this group variably cross-react in indirect immunofluorescent tests, and to a lesser extent in complement-fixation tests, but not in neutralization tests.

Stability and resistance

Despite the extensive work carried out on the biophysical and biochemical properties of this group of viruses, particularly on LCM and Pichinde viruses, there is very little published information regarding their stability or resistance. They are known to be susceptible to lipid solvents, reflecting their enveloped structure, to low pH and to irradiation, and Bowen[102] has confirmed the susceptibility of Lassa virus itself to ether, B-propiolactone and ultra-violet irradiation. He has also shown that it is relatively heat-resistant requiring a temperature of 60° for a full 60 minutes to completely inactivate a suspension containing 10^6 TCID 50/ml in tissue culture fluid containing 10 per cent calf serum.

The general stability of the arenaviruses under a variety of natural conditions, however, does not appear to have been investigated. There is, for instance, no information on their resistance to drying, their survival under varying conditions of temperature and humidity, their survival in shed blood, in urine or on fomites. Similarly, there is no actual information regarding the inactivation of the viruses by commonly used disinfectants. In the absence of such information it is presumed, as in the case of Hepatitis B, that the virus of Lassa fever will be inactivated by standard procedures using formaldehyde, gluteraldehyde and sodium hypochlorite, and recommendations for disinfection and decontamination have been based on these assumptions.

Antigenic constitution and relationships

The arenaviruses have been found to possess three distinct antigenic components responsible for stimulating antibodies: reacting by neutralization, Complement Fixation (CF) and Fluorescent Antibody Tests (FAT). Neutralization reactions are highly specific to the individual viruses but the other two reactions reveal antigenic affinities within the group, more cross-reactions occurring with the FAT reaction than by CF. The latter test, depending upon the reactions of a soluble antigen component, reveals relationships between most of the viruses of the group to form the so-called 'Tacaribe complex' including the Junin and Machupo viruses, but excluding LCM and Lassa virus. These last two appear to be highly specific in their reactions although some cross-reaction has been detected between them using the FAT reaction.

In Lassa virus there is a suggestion that the strains from

Sierra Leone and Nigeria may not be antigenically identical.[76, 79]

Mutability

There is as yet no evidence of mutability in respect to Lassa virus. There has been some suggestion that the behaviour of the virus may be different in Sierra Leone from Nigeria but there appears to be little justification for this idea. The only real evidence of difference lies in the lack of complete reciprocal neutralization, observed in one experiment, between virus strains and sera from the two areas.[76]

The issue of mutability is however of crucial importance, since a change in virus tropism in the human body could lead to a dramatic increase in the potential for person-to-person spread of infection. The low degree of infectiousness of patients during the early stages of the disease despite the presence of virus in the pharyngeal secretions and the constancy of cough as an early feature, has already been discussed (see p 97), and Monath[79] has suggested that the observation that only certain patients are infectious may be related to the concentration of virus in the throat. Lack of person-to-person transmission of Rubella vaccine virus has been explained on the same grounds. The facts suggest that there is a threshold concentration below which the presence of virus in the throat represents only a minimal hazard, even when the patient is suffering from a persistent cough.

It is impossible at present to surmise at what concentration a patient would become dangerous but it seems clear that an enhancement of respiratory tropism on the part of the virus could transform the situation from the present state of low transmissibility to one more closely comparable to that of influenza. A hint regarding the possible consequences can be found in the Zorzor episode. That the pneumonic presentation of the index case was not due to a pneumotropic mutation of the virus is evident from the lack of tertiary cases, but the ease of inducement of pneumotropism, with progressive enhancement of virus replication and case-fatality rate, by the simple process of lung passage is easily demonstrated in the laboratory with influenza virus and the devastating consequences in nature may be seen in the 1918–19 influenza pandemic.

Knowledge of the stability of the Lassa virus genome is critical to the development of a rational public health response.

Pathogenesis of infection

Portals of entry

The virus is capable of invading the body by a variety of routes depending upon the circumstances of contact. The only clearly proven route is that of direct inoculation as a result of hospital accident. The other routes are identified only through a study of the epidemiology of the disease. The probable portals of entry can be seen in Table 6.

TABLE 6   Portals of entry for Lassa fever

Portal of entry	Source of infection
Community-acquired infection	
Respiratory tract and/or conjunctiva	Rodent excreta
	Possibly respiratory tract of human cases
Alimentary tract	Food contaminated by rodent excreta
Possibly direct inoculation	Ectoparasites
Hospital-acquired infection	
Alimentary tract	Infected patients – heavy contamination through close contact
	Blood and infected body fluids
Respiratory tract and/or conjunctiva	Infected patients – close contact with droplet transmission
	Tracheostomy aerosols
	Autopsy exposure
Direct inoculation	Autopsy accidents
	Skin abrasions
	Syringe-needle accidents

Replication sites and distribution of virus

The virus is generalized throughout the body from an early stage of the disease and probably replicates in most tissues. Experimental investigations in animals and titration of autopsy specimens from human cases suggest that the concentrations of the virus in lungs, liver, kidney and spleen are higher than in the blood, while clinical and microscopic evidence indicates the presence of lesions in most tissues studied, including the pharynx and mycardium.[55] The evidence suggests that the virus is pantropic and probably multiplies freely in the reticuloendothelial system, probably including the bonemarrow, although there may be considerable species variation as suggested by the pathology of the disease in man and animals.[93]

In the presumptive rodent reservoir, *Mastomy natalensis*, widespread infection is produced without clinical signs of disease and the virus persists in many tissues and the urine for prolonged periods of time.[79] Since the virus is widely distributed in the body, all body fluids, including serous effusions and exudates, are highly infective.

In the guinea-pig, virus concentrations in the tissues reach $10^5 - 10^7$/g with a level of about one log lower in the blood. In the squirrel monkey and in neonatal *Mastomys natalensis*, the corresponding levels were about $10^{3.5} - 10^6$ and in adult *Mastomys* $10^{2.5} - 10^4$.[93]

Spread through the body

The high concentration of virus in the blood and the ability of the virus to infect following direct inoculation through the skin suggests that generalization is by haematogenous spread.

Shedding from the body

The two most obvious routes of virus shedding from an infected patient are from the pharynx and in the urine, the pharynx being the more dangerous. Intestinal haemorrhage, in association with diarrhoea and vomiting, may also lead to gross environmental contamination. Major haemorrhage may also occur from the vagina, particularly in pregnant women.

Infectious period

Theoretically, the infectious period of Lassa fever extends from the first appearance of virus in the pharyngeal secretions at, or shortly after, onset until final clearance of virus from the pharynx and urine, which may take several weeks. In practice, however, transmission appears to be limited to the height of the illness from about the sixth day after onset until death or clinical recovery – i.e. from the time of onset of severe ulcerative pharyngitis to termination of viraemia. No episodes of infection have been traced to residual viruria.

Vehicles of transfer of infection

The obvious vehicles of transfer of infection are:

pharyngeal secretions
urine
blood
body fluids and tissues
blood-stained excreta or vomit

These may act either through direct contamination of contacts or through freshly contaminated fomites such as swabs, bed-linen or utensils. The resistance of virus to drying has not been determined so the duration of infectivity of contaminated fomites is unknown. All pathological specimens are potentially or actually infective.

Clinical factors

Management

Gravely ill patients who suffer severe pharyngeal and abdominal pain which is associated with vomiting and diarrhoea and who require continued pharyngeal or tracheostomy care will present major problems in clinical management and isolation technique. The requirements for monitoring laboratory investigations, and supportive radiological or surgical intervention will also affect decisions regarding the type of isolation facilities adopted. These, however, are clinical issues outside the scope of this study.

Prophylaxis and therapy

Upecific prophylaxis is not at present available so general therapy is limited to nursing care and supportive measures. Measures to control the haemorrhagic tendency have not been particularly successful so far and it is unlikely that surgical intervention could be effective for the control of actual haemorrhages once the haemorrhagic tendency has developed.

Specific therapy is limited to the use of immune plasma or serum obtained from convalescent patients. The recovery of Dr Jordi Casals was attributed to such therapy, although its effectiveness is not proven.

The use of interferon in large doses may provide another therapeutic approach.

A recent report[90] of successful treatment of experimental infection in monkeys suggests that Ribavirin may be an effective therapeutic agent.

Overall conclusion

The final impression of Lassa fever which emerges from this study is of a dangerous virus zoonosis of a high lethality for man but it has little potential for person-to-person spread and negligible epidemic potential when the rodent reservoir is absent or not in very close association with human habitation.

The disease is probably an ancient one in West Africa with a normally low incidence in the human population punctuated by epidemics secondary to epizootic spread of infection in the rodent reservoir. It is likely that in the past there have been many unrecognized introductions of the disease into susceptible communities both in and out of Africa without producing secondary cases.

In hospital the disease represents a dangerous nosocomial hazard with a high case-fatality rate but low communicability. Its transmission usually requires close patient contact and many hospital-acquired cases are traceable to accident or to poor technique. Respiratory transmission is a clear possibility but rarely occurs.

No known instance of transmission has occurred outside Africa despite transporting patients at the height of their illness in commercial flights, nursing them under widely different degrees of isolation in hospitals of widely different levels of sophistication. The apparent low degree of communicability of the disease encourages the conclusion that it may be safely contained by applying standard nursing procedures under standard conditions of hospital isolation.

The main problem of containment lies in protection of the health care staff attending the patient.

7

Marburg Virus Disease

Epidemiology

1. History and analysis of outbreaks

Between 8 August and 10 September 1967, 30 cases of a previously unknown and highly lethal disease occurred as an explosive epidemic which affected three locations in continental Europe: Marburg, Frankfurt and Belgrade. A thirty-first case occurred on 8 November. Seven of the primary cases died but no deaths occurred among the secondary cases.[123-6]

The location of the cases is shown in Table 7 below.

TABLE 7   **The number and distribution of cases in the Marburg disease outbreak in 1967**
(modified from Martini 1971[125])

Location	Primary		Secondary (Nosocomial)		Secondary (Late)	
	Number	Fatal	Number	Fatal	Number	Fatal
Marburg	20	5	2	—	1	—
Frankfurt	4	2	2	—	—	—
Belgrade	1	—	1	—	—	—
Totals	25	7	5	—	1	—

The first alert occurred when three patients with alarming symptoms were admitted to the University Hospital, Marburg, during the third week of August by which time the first case, who died two days later, had already been nursed at home for two weeks.

During the two-week period between 14 and 27 August, 24 of the original 30 cases occurred, 22 of them were laboratory or animal-care workers who handled monkeys, their tissues or tissue-culture derivatives for virus vaccine production. This monkey association was rapidly appreciated but the disease was first thought to be a particularly severe form of dysentery – an impression which was speedily corrected when the characteristic symptomatology and course of the disease, and its failure to respond to antibiotic treatment, became clear.

The drastic measures that were taken with the suspect monkeys together with stringent protective measures for the staff brought the occurrence of laboratory-acquired infections to an abrupt halt although five secondary infections occurred among the medical and nursing staff attending the primary cases. Infection did not spread to the community and only two cases occurred among the patients' families. One was the wife of the single case in Belgrade and the second was the wife of a patient who was later found to have the virus in his semen and transmitted the infection during intercourse.[123] After this last case no further infections occurred and the disease disappeared.

During the following years a serological survey was carried out in Uganda by Henderson and his colleagues from CDC, Atlanta,[116] and antibodies were shown to be present in up to 36 per cent of vervet monkeys tested, with rising antibody titres in nine monkeys trapped in one area. Positive findings were also reported by Kalter[120] on a wide range of primate sera. In addition, three monkey trappers from Uganda were found to have antibodies, although these apparently positive results were later discounted. The antigen used in these studies was a relatively crude preparation of guinea-pig liver supplied by CDC and later work indicated that the positive results were due to non-specific reactions.[137]

At the same time it was shown that both vervet and rhesus monkeys were highly susceptible to infection by the virus and suffered a high mortality under experimental conditions.[115, 131, 132] This made it most unlikely that the vervet monkey could be the natural reservoir of the virus in Africa and did not support the concept of a widespread enzootic infection of the vervet population without a high death rate being noted. Moreover, with vervets being exported from Uganda at the rate of about 1,000 a month it did not seem possible that a virus of such virulence would not have been detected if it was indeed seeded through the monkey population to the extent suggested by the serological surveys.

The course of events during the outbreak strongly suggested that the vervet monkeys themselves had become infected from some external source during the period captivity prior to transport. The source was not discovered and all trace of the virus vanished until February 1975 when an Australian on vacation in Southern Africa contracted the infection while hiking in Rhodesia and died in Johannesburg.[112] His female companion and a young nurse who cared for them both also contracted the disease but recovered. Despite extensive investigations by Conrad of CDC,[108] the source of the virus was not traced. The only possible clue to the origin of the student's infection was that he was bitten or stung on the upper arm by an unidentified insect at about the time that he contracted the disease.

This second episode of Marburg virus infection showed clearly that the virus was not confined to Uganda but gave no indication of its origin, presumed animal reservoir, or its mode of transmission. The virus again vanished from sight and remained undetected until, in 1976, a closely related virus caused the highly lethal outbreaks of haemorrhagic fever in Sudan and Zaire (see page 117).

Clinical summary

The illness was characterized by an incubation period of three to eight days and abrupt onset with prostration, headache, generalized muscle pains and fever. Vomiting and watery diarrhoea developed during the next few days, the severity and persistence of the diarrhoea paralleled the severity of the illness. Pharyngitis and conjunctivitis occurred in most patients. Genital involvement with irritation and inflammation of the scrotum or labia majora was frequent and orchitis occurred in some patients. About the fifth day a maculo-papular rash developed with petaechiae in haemorrhagic cases. A haemorrhagic diatheses was apparent from about the eighth to the thirteenth day and was characterized by bleeding from the gums, intestine, vagina and urinary tract. After about the fifth day hepatitis and renal involvement developed which were followed by signs of myocarditis from about day 13. An early leucopaenia was followed by leucocytosis while thrombocytopaenia was present from about the third day onwards.

The peak of the illness occurred around the eighth to tenth day after which the fever slowly subsided with a secondary rise occurring between the twelfth and fourteenth day. Four cases died on the eighth and ninth days of illness and three on days 15, 16 and 17.

In surviving patients there was a marked loss of weight and recovery was slow with prostration persisting for many weeks. A number of patients suffered long-term sequelae including hepatitis, orchitis, myelitis, psychosis and mental disability. The persistence of atypical mononuclear cells, given the term 'virucytes', in the blood of some patients raised the suspicion of persistent or latent infection. This occurred in one patient and was inadvertently proven when his wife became venereally infected with the virus three months after the patient's own illness. The virus was subsequently isolated from his semen.

Convalescent serum from early cases was used in the treatment of some of the later patients and was felt to have modified the course of the illness in them.

A full account of the clinical picture of the disease together with its diagnosis and management may be found in the monograph 'Marburg Virus Disease',[123] in the account by Gear *et al.*[112] of the Johannesburg episode and in the WHO publication 'Marburg and Ebola Virus Infections: A Guide for their Diagnosis, Management and Control' by Simpson.[133]

Analysis of outbreaks

Human infections. In all the primary human cases there was a clear-cut association with vervet monkeys of two particular batches in Germany and three in Belgrade. Twenty of the 25 primary cases had carried out procedures involving direct contact with monkey tissues and blood. These included surgical procedures such as the removal of kidneys and brains, opening the thorax and abdomen, autopsies and taking blood samples. Although gloves, gowns and masks were supposed to be worn for all operative procedures it is not clear to what extent this was done but it is certain that such precautions were not conscientiously applied. For instance, three of the four primary cases in Frankfurt had removed kidneys without wearing gloves.[135]

Direct contamination with blood had occurred in all the primary cases of this group.[123]

Of the remaining five primary cases three had been cleaning tissue culture containers set up from the infected monkeys, one had broken a tissue culture flask containing infected material and one had been mincing and trypsinizing infected kidney tissue.

The sources of infection of the five original secondary cases were equally obvious: two were physicians who had pricked themselves with syringe needles after taking blood from infected patients; one was an autopsy attendant who assisted at the autopsy of one of the fatal cases and contaminated his forearms with blood; one was a nurse who cared for patients in the hospital at Marburg and the last was the wife of the single primary case at Belgrade, a veterinarian who had performed four autopsies on dead monkeys. This patient nursed her husband and had direct contact with his blood on the fourth and fifth days of his illness when she handled bloodstained bedlinen.[123]

The sixth and final secondary case occurred as the result of venereal transmission in the wife of one of the primary cases three months after the latter's illness.[123] The types of exposure are summarized in Table 8.

TABLE 8   Types of contact exposure
(Modified from Hennessen 1971[117])

Exposure	Number of cases	Number of fatal cases
Surgical procedures with monkeys	20	5
Cleaning contaminated tissue culture containers	3	1
Trypsinization and mincing of monkey tissues	1	1
Accident – broken tissue culture flask	1	—
Patient contact – syringe needle accident	2	—
Patient contact – nursing	2	—
Autopsy contamination with blood	1	– –
Venereal	1	—

While it is not possible to identify the precise route of infection in the majority of the original cases, they clearly all involved very close direct contact and 20 of the primary cases experienced direct contamination with blood from infected monkeys. In no instance was there evidence of remote transmission.

Source of infection

Investigation of the history of the vervet monkeys which were the immediate source of the infection showed that they reached Germany in two batches on 21 and 28 July, and Belgrade in three batches on 18 and 23 July and 1 August. The monkeys arriving in Germany were used within a short space of time while those reaching Belgrade were placed in quarantine for a period of six weeks before use. During this period, they suffered an abnormally high mortality as shown in Table 9.

TABLE 9   **Mortality among three batches of monkeys in Belgrade from August–September 1967**
(Modified from Hennessen 1971[117])

Monkey batch	Date delivered	Number	Deaths to 7 September	Mortality (in %)
I	18 August	99	45	45
II	23 August	95	20	21
III	1 September	94	30	32

The single human case occurring in Belgrade was a veterinarian who carried out four autopsies in animals which died late in this quarantine period during the last week of August. Epidemiological analysis[123] seemed to indicate that infection had been introduced into these batches of monkeys before their arrival in continental Europe. This occurred either during a 9–36 hour staging stop at London Airport where they were in contact with some 48 species of different animals, or during the previous three days when they were held in captivity in Uganda. It seemed clear that in either event, spread of infection had occurred during transportation and after arrival. It seems most likely that the origin of the infection did in fact lie within Africa and this conclusion is strongly supported by the subsequent events in South Africa and, later, in Sudan and Zaire.

Several workers have now found that the virus is highly lethal to monkeys. Simpson *et al.* at Porton[131-2] and Haas and Maas in Germany[115] found 100 per cent mortality in vervet, rhesus and squirrel monkeys even with very small inocula. This lethality makes it unlikely that the vervet monkey is the primary reservoir of the virus and suggests that it acted as an amplifying reservoir for the human outbreak. The ambiguity in the interpretation of the serological survey results has already been discussed and it is now generally agreed that no indication of the source of the virus has yet been detected.

2. Case-fatality rate

Seven deaths occurred among the 25 primary cases giving a case-fatality rate of 28 per cent. The overall case-fatality rate was 23 per cent since all the secondary cases recovered. This recovery may have been due to the use of convalescent serum in their treatment, it is also likely that a smaller virus dosage may have been involved. Table 10 shows the results obtained by Haas and Maas in a titration of infective serum from a moribund monkey. While the serum was shown to produce lethal infection at the remarkably high dilution of 10^{-10} the prolongation of survival time above the 10^{-6} level is clear-cut. In an infection which was not uniformly lethal such amelioration of severity would show as a reduction in fatality rate.

TABLE 10 **Marburg virus: Time of death of vervet monkey inoculated with various dilutions of first passage blood from a vervet monkey inoculated from a patient**
(Modified from Haas and Maas[115])

Inoculum dilution	Time of death (days pot-infection)
10^0	5, 7
10^{-2}	7, 7, 6
10^{-4}	7, 9
10^{-6}	8, 10, 10
10^{-8}	11, 12
10^{-10}	14, 25

3. Community incidence

4. Seasonal incidence

5. Ecology

Apart from these two incidents there is no known human incidence of Marburg disease and no knowledge regarding its ecology although it seems certain that an animal reservoir must exist.

6. Vector requirements

By analogy with the many arbovirus infections which exist in Africa, it is likely that an arthropod vector may prove to be involved in transmitting the infection in nature. While this is currently a matter of speculation it may be significant that multiplication of the virus in one mosquito species, *Aedes aegypti*, has been experimentally demonstrated.[123] Multiplication did not occur in the one Anopheles species tested (*Anopheles maculipennis*).

7. Mechanisms of transmission

With the exception of the index case in South Africa, all human infections so far have involved close physical contact with infective material, in most cases the blood of infected monkeys or patients. Apart from the two episodes of needle accidents, the precise portals of entry cannot be identified but clearly skin abrasions, ocular and oral contamination or heavy droplet respiratory infection could be involved. Haas and Maas[115] found that infection was transmitted to caged monkeys when these were *immediately adjacent* within mutual touching distance but not when they were separated by a distance of 1–2 m. Other workers have, however, found that monkeys in the same room are liable to infection even at a distance.[131] Despite ample opportunity, no case of remote transmission occurred in the two human outbreaks. Transmission among monkeys within the animal quarters was certainly mediated by the attendant staff.

8. Infectious period of the patient

The infectious period of the patient cannot be precisely judged from present information. Siegert and Slenczka[129] detected virus in only two of six throat washings and one of four urines taken at the acute stage of the disease and found it to be on the borderline of detectability. Five stool specimens were found to be negative. These findings suggest that virus is not shed from the body in any great quantity, despite the clinical evidence of pharyngitis, unless haemorrhage occurs. Clearly, any blood-stained material will be highly infectious by direct contact.

Since the virus will presumably be generalized in even the earliest stages of the illness, blood and all laboratory specimens must be regarded as infectious from the onset. There is no indication of infection during the incubation period. A specific hazard appears to exist in relation to genital carriage during convalescence. Genital symptoms with irritation and inflammation of the external genitalia and, in a few patients, orchitis, were noted during the outbreak. In one case, following an episode of venereal transmission, virus was isolated twice from the semen of the primary patient up to three months after the time of his infection.[123] Similar convalescent carriage in the semen was demonstrated following recovery from Ebola virus infection in a laboratory worker at MRE (Porton[111]). The presence of 'virucytes' in the blood of a few patients during late convalescence also suggests the possibility of long-term carriage or latent infection following clinical recovery.

9. Transmissibility

Transmissibility of the disease is clearly of a very low order, despite its danger to medical personnel attending patients.

From the figures given by Martini[125] and Hennessen[117] it is evident that the first case to occur in Marburg was nursed at home for two weeks before admission to hospital two days before his death, and that, between them, the next 22 cases spent a total of 93 days in the community between onset of illness and admission to hospital. In spite of these extended opportunities for contact, no secondary cases occurred in the community. Of the four nosocomial secondary cases in Germany only one was due to patient contact, two were caused by needle pricks and one by direct contamination with blood at autopsy.

In the one secondary case in Belgrade direct contact with blood was also known to have occurred during nursing. It is also significant that in Belgrade a total of 95 monkeys died over a period of 50 days. It is not possible to say how many were due to Marburg virus infection, but the fact that the veterinarian who carried out autopsies towards the end of this chain of deaths contracted the infection suggests that the virus must have been propagated in the colony during that period. Despite this, no infection occurred among the animals' attendants, and in Germany the staff who attended the animals at night and weekends, but did no operative work, did not become infected.

The index case in the South African episode was followed by a secondary infection in his female companion who had been in close contact with him throughout and by a further case in the nurse who had nursed him during the last two nights of his illness when he was suffering from severe vomiting and watery diarrhoea, both being heavily bloodstained. During the first two hours she was on duty the nurse did not wear protective clothing. After his death the nurse attempted to console his girlfriend while the girlfriend was coming down with the disease. It is not clear from which contact the nurse derived her infection.

This episode is particularly interesting because of the formidable array of laboratory investigations which were carried out on all three cases to establish the diagnosis and guide management.[112] Although the diagnosis of Marburg infection was not made until the third case had been ill for four days and the second case for thirteen, Lassa fever was suspected when the first case died and full precautions were immediately taken. Despite this, the clinical management of the two remaining patients was continued with full monitoring of the blood picture and biochemistry and with the investigations carried out in the hospital diagnostic laboratory.

The overall picture which emerges from these two outbreaks of Marburg virus infection is that of a highly dangerous disease of very limited transmissibility and no suggestion of epidemic potential in the community.

EBOLA FEVER

The greater part of the information relating to Ebola fever in Sudan and Zaire has been derived from the World Health Organization Report, 1978, Bull, WHO *56*: 245–294, from 'Ebola Virus Haemorrhagic Fever'. Proceedings of an International Colloquium on Ebola Virus Infection and Other Haemorrhagic Fevers held in Antwerp, Belgium, 6–8 December 1977, and by personal discussion with Dr Karl Johnson, Dr Stanley Foster, Dr S. R. Pattyn, Dr D. I. H. Simpson and Dr G. van der Groen.

Most of the information on the laboratory behaviour of the virus was obtained in personal discussion with Dr E. T. W. Bowen and from his comprehensive Ph.D. thesis.[102]

8

Ebola Fever

Epidemiology

1. History and analysis of outbreaks

During the second half of 1976 there were two contemporaneous outbreaks of haemorrhagic fever with high mortality in central Africa. The two areas affected were, first the southern Sudan where the epidemic started on 27 June and lasted until 20 November causing 284 known cases and 151 deaths for a case-fatality rate of 53 per cent. The second area was northeastern Zaire where the first known case occurred on 1 September and the last on 24 October. In Zaire there were 318 known cases and 280 deaths with only 38 serologically confirmed recoveries. The case-fatality rate in this epidemic was 88 per cent – the highest ever recorded for any virus infection other than rabies. A second epidemic in the same region of the southern Sudan occurred between July and October 1979. Out of a total of 33 confirmed cases, 22 deaths resulted for a case-fatality rate of 67 per cent.

The World Health Organization was requested for assistance in September and organized two separate teams to investigate the two outbreaks.

Clinical summary

The disease was very similar in its clinical manifestations in both localities, although the Zaire epidemic showed a considerably higher case-fatality rate. Onset was sudden with headache, muscle and joint pains and fever. The disease developed as a progressively more severe influenza-like illness until by the seventh day the patient was prostrated with deeply sunken eyes and a ghost-like, expressionless face. Chest pain, often pleuritic in nature, accompanied by a dry cough developed early and was followed in the second week by diarrhoea, first watery, then bloodstained, and frequently by vomiting. The gastrointestinal symptoms were accompanied by severe cramping abdominal pains. In patients who recovered the vomiting and diarrhoea lasted about seven days but the abdominal pain might continue for several weeks.

Dryness of the mouth and throat were sometimes extreme, but true pharyngitis did not appear to be a feature of the disease. A morbilliform skin rash was sometimes seen around the fifth day and was followed by desquamation.

A haemorrhagic diathesis with cutaneous and subconjunctival haemorrhages and frank bleeding from any or all body orifices was common; it was present in 91 per cent of fatal cases and about 50 per cent of the non-fatal ones. Mental derangement was also frequently seen and, in recovered cases, sometimes persisted into convalescence. In fatal cases death usually occurred around the sixth to eighth day of illness and convalescence was very slow in recovered cases.

In Zaire, respiratory symptoms were less frequently seen than in the Sudanese outbreak.

Analysis of outbreaks

Sudan epidemics.[128b] Investigation determined that the Sudan epidemic had originated in a cotton factory in the township of Nzara near the southern border of the country. The factory, employing about 455 workers, was part of an agricultural cooperative of some 2,000 employees in a district with a total population of about 20,000.

Between 27 June and 18 July 1976, three factory employees developed acute haemorrhagic fever and died. Detailed investigation suggested that these three men had been infected independently. The first two cases each gave rise to only one secondary case of which one died, but the third case started a chain of infection which resulted in 48 cases and 27 deaths. All of these cases were infected by direct close contact with sick patients, usually involving nursing and patient care.

The apparent requirement for close direct contact for transmission to occur made the tracing of sources of infection relatively easy. Despite this, 14 cases were identified in Nzara,

9 of them among factory employees, where no such contact with sick persons could be determined. It was suspected that some of these represented primary infections from some unknown source. The Nzara outbreak burned itself out before the end of October without intervention.

From Nzara, infection was introduced into Maridi, a town of some 10,000 inhabitants 180 km to the east, ón 7 August and again on 29 August by the admission of two patients from Nzara to the Maridi hospital, a busy training institution for nurses with a staff of 230.

The first of these cases infected four close contacts, a close friend, a nurse, a hospital cleaner and a hospital messenger, all of whom assisted in looking after him during the 10 days in hospital before he died. These new cases were in turn admitted to various wards in the hospital and each infected a further series of close contacts including visitors who seeded the infection into the town of Maridi. Within the hospital, the cycle of infection continued. Staff caring for patients transferred the infection to other patients and themselves became infected, to be in their turn admitted to serve as further foci of infection. Visitors who helped in nursing the patients also continued to become infected and continued seeding the town community. Finally, as the population became aware that the hospital was the focal point of the epidemic, patients were removed by their relatives to their own homes and further spread the infection through the town. During this period 93 of Maridi's 213 cases acquired their disease in the hospital, 72 were hospital staff who became infected while carrying out their duties. Forty-one per cent of the student nurses became infected.

By contrast with Nzara where the hospital was small and admitted few patients for short periods of time, the Maridi hospital acted as an amplifier of the epidemic and the source of the community infection.

Intervention by the Sudanese health authorities who established isolation premises within the hospital, distribution of protective clothing and the adoption of basic barrier-nursing techniques, appeared to reduce the incidence of infection in the early part of October, but cases increased again towards the end of the month when the supply of protective clothing ran out. The situation was finally controlled only after the arrival of the

WHO team on 29 October when adequate protective clothing was available and strict training in its use and in decontamination and barrier-nursing procedures was instituted.

The epidemic in the community was also brought under control by an intensive surveillance campaign using locally recruited teams of volunteers to locate all cases of infection in the town and its environs with a view to their admission to hospital isolation. In spite of a number of refusals of admission these containment measures were successful and no further cases occurred after the end of November.

During the height of the epidemic in late September two cases were transferred to the regional hospital in Juba where one nurse became infected, and two travelled to Khartoum, 1,000 km north, where they died in hospital without causing secondary infections.

The disappearance of the disease at the end of the epidemic appeared complete, and no evidence of an animal reservoir was found even among bats and other rodents captured in the cotton factory; nor was there any evidence of persistent human carriage. Three years later, in late July 1979, a 45-year-old man from the Nzara area fell ill, was admitted to the Nzara Hospital and died within three days with gross haemorrhagic manifestations. A patient in the next bed and a visitor became infected and died and there were two further cases in the hospital staff. From the hospital, infection again spread to the community and initiated an epidemic lasting two months, the last known case being on 6 October. There was a total of 33 confirmed cases, 22 died, giving a case-fatality rate of 67 per cent.

In a limited serological survey, it was found that about 6 per cent of 203 members of the Nzara population was serologically positive for anti-Ebola antibody, suggesting that the virus is in fact endemic or enzootic in the area.

The epidemic again followed the 1976 pattern in that the hospital acted as the amplifying system through which the community epidemic was initiated and again it was clear that very close contact – such as nursing the sick patients or preparing bodies for burial – was necessary for transmission of infection. Casual contact was not sufficient for transmission to occur.

Zaire epidemic.[128c] The Zaire epidemic started, as far as could be determined, with a single case whose onset was on 1 September; like the Maridi epidemic; it was hospital mediated although in a different manner.

Yambuku, with its mission hospital 'YMH' which was the epicentre of the outbreak, lies north of the Zaire River in the extreme north of the country about 900 km from the Sudan border and Nzara to the east.

Between 1 September and 24 October, 318 known cases occurred with 280 deaths within a 120 km radius of Yambuku in the Bumba Zone of the Equateur Region. This region is predominantly rural with three-quarters of its population of 275,000 living in villages which are mostly of fewer than 500 persons. Half of the population is under 15 years of age. Two additional cases occurred in the capital Kinshasa, 1,500 km southwest of the region.

The Yambuku Catholic Mission, with its hospital, is one of seven in the Bumba Zone. The mission is about 100 km north of Bumba and is the principle source of health care for a population of about 60,000 persons in the Yandongi and adjacent collectivities. In 1976 it had 120 beds and a staff of 17 including a Zairian medical assistant and three Belgian nursing sisters. It also had a very active out-patient clinic which included pre-natal and obstetrical services and treated between 6,000 and 12,000 patients every month.

Each morning the nursing staff were issued with five syringes and needles of various sizes to use in the out-patient clinics. These syringes were not sterilized during the day but in between patients they were rinsed in a pan of warm water; sometimes at the end of the day they were boiled.

The surgical theatre had its own supply of syringes and instruments which were autoclaved after use.

Origin and course of the epidemic

The first known case was a 44-year-old instructor at the mission school who had toured northern Equateur by car with six other instructors during 8–22 August. When he returned on 22 August he developed a fever which was diagnosed as malaria and, on 26 August, was given a chloroquin injection at the out-patient clinic. His fever promptly subsided but recurred five days later on 1 September. He became progressively worse and was admitted to the hospital on 5 September with gastrointestinal bleeding. He died on 8 September.

During that first week of September at least nine other cases occurred; all had received injections at the out-patient clinic. During the eight-week period to 24 October, 318 cases occurred with only 38 recoveries giving a case-fatality rate of 88 per cent.

During the course of the epidemic 55 of the 250 villages within 120 km of Yambuku were affected. The highest attack rate was in the Yandongi collectivity immediately surrounding Yambuku where 43 of 73 villages were involved and the attack rate was 8 per 1,000 of the population as compared with less than 2 per 1,000 in the six other collectivities.

Most of the villages had few cases, 85 per cent had fewer than 10 cases each and only three villages (6 per cent) had 20 or more. During the first two weeks all cases were restricted to within 30 km of Yambuku.

Thirteen of the 17 members of the YMH staff contracted the disease and 11 of them died. The hospital closed on 3 October. From that time there was no medical intervention but for some reason the epidemic burned itself out by 24 October before the arrival of the WHO team.

During this period, however, on 25 September, one of the YMH nursing sisters, in the third day of her illness, was flown to Kinshasa and admitted to the Ngaliema Hospital where she died five days later. A second nursing sister, who had accompanied her from Yambuku and nursed her in Kinshasa without protective clothing, became ill on 8 October and died on 14 October. On the 13 October a third nurse, from the Ngaliema Hospital, fell ill and died on 20 October.

This third case was of special significance since it was the first infection to have occurred indisputably in Kinshasa and the circumstances of its occurrence were extremely alarming. This nurse had cared for the first sister, who arrived ill from Yambuku, but *not* for the second who became ill on 8 October. In the interim she went on leave from the hospital during the incubation period of the illness, and for the first few days after onset, she lived with her family and was active in arranging an overseas study leave. She therefore generated a large number of contacts in the community including numerous officials at the

Ministry of Foreign Affairs. Among the close contacts was her young brother. She shared a snack meal with him two days after the onset of symptoms and the day before her admission to hospital she and her brother both drank from the same bottle of pop. This situation caused a near panic in Kinshasa with its population of two million and also meant that the incubation period of the disease could extend to 21 days, causing an uncomfortable prolongation of quarantine periods.

Until her death on 20 October, this nurse was cared for by her sister, also a nurse. By this time, at the request of the Zaire Government, Dr Margaret Isaacson arrived from South Africa with Marburg immune plasma and took charge of isolation and quarantine precautions at the hospital. The nurse looking after the third patient was given protective clothing and rapidly trained in barrier nursing technique. She refused, however, to wear a full-face protective mask. The courage of this nurse was remarkable as she nursed her sister until her death, and then waited through a full three-week period while all of Kinshasa waited for her to fall ill and die. Since further cases were expected a plastic isolator from the Canadian government was flown in to the hospital and personnel were trained to use it by Sgt Colbourne of the National Defence Medical Centre in Ottawa.

Dr Isaacson's precautions proved effective however and no further cases occurred. The quarantined nurse and medical staff from the relevant ward of the hospital together with primary contacts outside the hospital who were brought in by the authorities were released from quarantine at the end of the 21-day period. Particularly significant is the fact that the nurse's young brother, who she shared the bottle of 'pop' with two days after the onset of her illness, did not contract the disease.

The control of this threatening situation in Kinshasa was the first concern of the WHO team and until it was achieved they were not free to proceed with surveillance in the primary epidemic area. The advance surveillance parties did not in fact reach Yambuku until 9 November and by the end of the month it had become clear that the last probable case had died on 5 November.

Clinical summary

Clinically the disease in Zaire closely resembled that in the Sudan, but there were certain differences. The most striking was that in Zaire the respiratory symptoms were less marked than in the Sudan, the case-fatality rate was higher – 88 per cent as compared with 53 per cent – and the incubation period in those cases which acquired infection by parenteral inoculation at the YMH was shorter than in those naturally infected. It seemed also that the disease in these cases tended to be even more severe. It was felt that these last two observations might be due to higher virus dosage and faster dissemination of the virus.

2. Case-fatality rate

Although the case-fatality rates were high in both the Sudan and Zaire outbreaks there was a marked difference between them. In the Sudan the overall rate was 53 per cent with little difference between Nzara and Maridi while in Zaire the rate was 88 per cent.

The reason for this difference has not been elucidated but two findings are significant. First, Bowen found a consistent difference between the Sudan and Zaire strains in their virulence in experimental infections: the Zaire strain is uniformly lethal to monkeys while the Sudan strain is not.[102] Second, Bowen also demonstrated adaptations of the Zaire strain to guinea pigs by serial passage. In the first pass, 9 out of 10 guinea pigs survived infection by the acute phase blood of a Zaire patient. In the next three passages the incubation period was slightly shortened and stabilized and the lethality of the infection rose to 100 per cent in the fourth passage.

The first observation supports the concept that the difference in lethality observed in the human epidemics was genuine and was referable to the virus rather than to the relative susceptibilities of the two human populations. The second indicates an adaptive potential on passage which could be equally applicable to serial human infections. Further work on the genetic stability of the virus is clearly required.

Inapparent infections

Both in the Sudan and in Zaire there was serological evidence of small numbers of minor or even sub-clinical infections. In Maridi it was found that in 64 members of the hospital staff, 7 (11 per cent) possessed antibody demonstrable by immuno-fluorescence; in 102 close family contacts, 20 were positive; and in 29 members of a school, tested as hopefully negative controls, 2 (7 per cent) were positive. These figures indicate about 17 per cent of sub-clinical infections among selected close contacts and a few among a more protected group.

In Zaire, detailed investigation in one village with a population of 415 showed 25 cases of clinical illness, an attack rate of 6 per cent, and 5 probable silent infections. In a wider survey of the epidemic area 2.4 per cent of 415 household contacts and 0.9 per cent of non-contacts were shown to have antibody without having had a febrile illness.

Although the incidence of sub-clinical infection was small, that they occurred at all is particularly interesting in that they occurred in a population which was presumed to have no pre-existing protective antibody against this virus.

3. Community incidence and mortality

There is no known endemic incidence of Ebola fever and consequently its mortality can be assessed only in relation to the two epidemic situations so far encountered.

In the Sudan, if the total population figures for the Maridi and Nzara areas are used for the calculation, the incidence was about 9 per 1,000, or about 2 per 1,000 per month, with a mortality of half those figures. However, the calculation has little meaning since there is no way of delimiting the population at risk. All that can be said with certainty is that, in the better defined area of Maridi, a little over 2 per cent of the population contracted the disease and a little over 1 per cent died of it.

In the more heavily exposed Yandongi collectivity of Zaire, the incidence was estimated at 8 per 1,000 compared with less than 2 per 1,000 in the six more peripheral collectivities, falling to zero 120 km from Yambuku.

It is important to realize that such figures have no value in assessing the possible impact of the disease if it was introduced into a Western community. At face value, the Maridi incidence would imply that the corresponding situation in a Western city, with a population of about 300,000, would result in 6,500 cases and about 3,500 deaths – an overwhelming disaster. However, the Maridi circumstances could not be even approximated in any city in any modern developed community.

Of greater value are the secondary and subsequent attack rates observed within definable contact groups such as families nursing sick patients since they apply to circumstances which represent, by Western standards, gross familial overcrowding and primitive living conditions and provide an acceptable upper limit to transmissibility which would not be matched in a developed community.

In Sudan, 36 families with 38 primary cases, were studied and secondary attack rates of 13, 14 and 9 per cent were observed for three generations of transmission, giving an average of 12 per cent. In Zaire, a similar study of 92 families in 21 villages gave contact attack rates of 16.7, 3.6, and 9 per cent, averaging 9.8 per cent for three successive generations. However, for 'families' defined as all persons living in contiguous housing and sharing common eating facilities, the secondary attack rate never exceeded 8 per cent.

In summary, it may be concluded that in both epidemics the secondary attack rate was in the region of 10 per cent. In the large and intimately associated family groups in Zaire, five generations of transmission were found in one instance and in Sudan, it was estimated that a total of 15 generations occurred in the entire community, but with the low attack rates, the epidemics were unable to maintain themselves even under primitive and overcrowded conditions.

4. Seasonal incidence

No seasonal incidence can be determined.

5. Ecology

Nothing is currently known about the ecology of the disease. In Zaire the origin of the epidemic remained a complete mystery.

The evidence strongly suggests that the first observed case of the disease was infected, like the others contracting the disease, during the first week of September by a contaminated malaria inoculation at the YMH. His two week trip through the northern forests seems to be irrelevant. If this is true, then the only hint to the possible mode of introduction of the virus is found in a brief record of a patient who had been admitted to the medical ward on 28 August with a diagnosis of 'dysentery and epistaxis'. This patient was removed from the hospital two days later and was never traced, apparently unknown to the residents and authorities of Yandongi.

In the absence of any suggestive evidence to guide such an investigation it was decided not to attempt to track down an animal reservoir in the area.

In the Sudan the situation was different. Here, despite the ease with which a source of infection could usually be identified for each case – for instance, sources were traced to identifiable contacts in all but five of 203 cases investigated in Maridi and in 53 of 67 cases in Nzara – there were 14 cases in Nzara for which no contact could be traced. Nine were employees of the cotton factory and six of them had worked in one particular area comprising the cloth room and adjacent store. Investigation of the habits and contacts of these cases suggested a strong likelihood that those occurring in the cotton factory employees were primary common source infections.

Among the possible animal reservoirs in the area the black rat *Rattus rattus* which infested the factory and an insectivorous bat, *Tadarida trevori*, which colonized the roof spaces in large numbers, seemed to be the most likely. Rodents and bats were collected from the cloth room vicinity of the cotton factory and blood and tissue samples were sent to Porton for virus isolation attempts. Not all the specimens have yet been processed, but so far no indication of infection has been obtained.

Although it seems likely, as in the case of the related Marburg virus, that infection was originally derived from an animal reservoir, there is still no clue as to what this reservoir might be.

6. Vector requirements

An African virus infection where the virus is present throughout the blood in high concentration and which is demonstrably transmissible by direct implantation is likely to be transmitted by biting arthropods. In Marburg virus, moreover, multiplication of the virus in *A. aegypti* has been demonstrated.[123] The limited surveys which have so far been conducted have failed to identify a mosquito vector. Other arthropods have not been investigated.

7. Mechanisms of infection

Apart from the route of direct implantation of virus, transmission has been strikingly dependent upon close direct physical contact, and there has been no evidence of transfer of infection from proximity alone. Sleeping in the same room was not sufficient, either in Sudan or Zaire, to achieve transfer, nor was any casual infection seen in passers-by or in contacts of primary contacts. The Sudan study team states: 'From these observations it is evident that nursing a patient was almost a requirement for becoming infected'.[128b]

While it is not possible to identify the precise route or mode of infection resulting from such close contact, the most probable route of transferring the virus is by the hands from a haemorrhaging patient to the mouth, nose or conjunctiva. Particularly important is that respiratory transmission did not appear to occur.

8. Infectious period of the patient

Virological studies in Ebola and Marburg virus infections have yielded no evidence of significant virus shedding by any route other than that of haemorrhage.

There appears to be little virus in the throat or urine but the persistence of virus in the seminal fluid[111, 123] poses a special risk of late venereal transmission. From the first day the blood contains a high concentration of virus which, in experimental monkeys, reaches a peak between the sixth and ninth days of illness and declines sharply after the appearance of detectable levels of circulating antibody. In the one human case where the viraemia was followed until the patient's death, the highest titre of virus was recorded on the seventh day, but high levels were observed throughout. In the case of the Porton scientist who suffered a laboratory infection, viraemia was detected at the level of $10^{4.5}$ guinea pig infectious units (GPIU)/ml within 14 hours of onset and persisted until the eighth day of illness, although the titre was reduced to $10^{0.5}$ GPIU/ml following immune plasma transfusion on the second day. The limited virological studies in man when taken in conjunction with the transmission pattern of the disease suggest that patients are not infectious during the incubation period or even in the early stages after onset of symptoms. This is supported particularly by the absence of transmission from the Zairian nurse on leave in Kanshasa during the incubation period despite the fact that she even shared a bottle of 'pop' with her younger brother after the onset of symptoms.

Infectivity appears to be dependent on haemorrhage and consequently parallels the bleeding tendency. It is mediated by infected blood itself or by bloodstained effluvia. Since viraemia develops rapidly, all diagnostic or pathological specimens must be regarded as infectious from onset or even before – this last statement is important with respect to blood samples taken from contacts under surveillance.

9. Transmissibility

Like Marburg disease, transmissibility of Ebola fever is clearly of a very low order – a fact repeated in the reports of the WHO teams and understandable from the natural history of the disease.

This assertion, however, does not appear to comply with the occurrence of a three-fold epidemic totalling at least 600 cases with over 400 deaths. The epidemic was triggered in Nzara by a small number of primary cases, in Maridi by only two introductions, and in Zaire by probably only one single undetected index case. A rational explanation is required and is found in the special circumstances in the epidemic areas – even here it was a different set of special circumstances which prevailed in the three epidemic regions. They must be closely studied if sound conclusions are to be made about the possibility of the circumstances recurring in a Western setting if the virus was inadvertently introduced, or, if any other circumstances more appropriate to developed communities could be envisaged which would lead to a similar result. The three episodes will, therefore, be separately considered.

Nzara. In Nzara out of a possible 14 primary cases where contacts could not be identified, 13 gave rise to only 5 secondary cases with no further transmission. This is in keeping with the low transmissibility of the disease. The remaining case PG, however, started a chain of infection which extended to 48 individuals. The remarkable results in this instance were apparently because he was a very gregarious, lively and popular character who was well-known in his neighbourhood. When he became ill, this popularity led to visits by a large number of friends, many of whom would have helped to care for him to some degree. It was through this unusually large number of close contacts that infection was so widely disseminated. It is important that, despite this dramatic start to the epidemic in Nzara, each succeeding case was traceable to a close direct contact and the outbreak burned itself out spontaneously without external intervention. There was, in this course of events, no suggestion that the chain of infection was due to the emergence of a virus variant with enhanced transmissibility, possibly by the respiratory route.

The special circumstances of this particular episode lie in the close exposure of a large number of people outside the patient's immediate family circle during the acute stage of his disease. This was clearly a rare event which was not duplicated in any other patient's case within the entire epidemic areas, nor would it be likely to occur in any developed community especially among the social strata likely to be exposed to infection and to introduce it to the country by air travel. It is also likely that the case in question would be hospitalized quickly so that exposure to visitors would be prevented.

Maridi. In Maridi the special circumstance was the role of the hospital as an amplifier of the infection once it had been introduced through the admission of two sick patients from Nzara. Isolating infectious patients was not practised in the hospital and there was no protective clothing for nurses, medical staff or visitors. The nurses, who were predominantly male, were usually dressed in short-sleeved shirts or singlets and short trousers which gave no protection to the heavy environmental contamination of haemorrhage, diarrhoea and vomiting which characterized the disease. Staff contracting the disease were admitted to various hospital wards where they formed fresh foci of infection. This self-replicating cycle resulted in infecting 72 members of 230 hospital staff. Out of the 213 cases in Maridi, 93 acquired their infections in the hospital (44 per cent).

The township community was rapidly infected from the hospital. Visitors customarily assisted in caring and feeding their relatives who were patients. If they became infected they constituted a channel through which the town was seeded. This initial seeding was soon reinforced as the extreme danger of the hospital environment was recognized and patients were removed by their relatives to their own homes.

Once dispersed in the community, however, the epidemic could not maintain itself for long with an intrafamilial transmission rate of only 12 per cent and virtually no transmission to outside contacts. It would have undoubtedly burnt itself out even without the prompt action of the WHO team who introduced protective clothing, isolation techniques in the hospital, together with effective surveillance, and case-finding in the community.

All the elements of the growth and spread of the epidemic in Maridi can be recognized as standard hazards of nosocomial infections and are well understood in modern hospital practice, even if their control is poorly executed in almost all of the hospitals. The operative elements were fourfold:

(1) transfer of infection to hospital staff as a result of poor nursing techniques;
(2) transfer of infection between hospitalized patients as for (1) and through the lack of patient isolation;
(3) infection of visitors through lack of elementary precautions and control, compounded in this instance by using visitors to help in patient care;
(4) the discharge or, in this instance, removal of infected patients from the hospital with the result of transferring the infection to the community.

On a more mundane scale each of these elements may be seen to operate almost daily with respect to staphylococcal infection in Western hospitals.

In spite of the ubiquity of these factors, it would be inconceivable that the Maridi situation could be paralleled in any hospital in a fully developed country. It is impossible to envisage this occurring in Western communities where the importance of hospital infection control has increased so markedly during the last few years, and where effective nursing techniques and isolation procedures have been developed precisely for the purpose of controlling highly communicable infections. It is possible that a first introduction will go unrecognized at the start and that full precautions will not be taken in time to prevent some transfer of infection within a hospital, but at the first alarm total isolation of the patient and full use of protective clothing and other measures by the staff would immediately check any further spread.

Zaire. In Zaire the epidemic was also hospital generated but in a different manner. The vector in this case was the outpatient clinic of the YMH with its unsterilized syringes where some 85 patients were seemingly inoculated directly with the virus. As in Maridi, once the epidemic was under way, the danger of the hospital environment was quickly recognized and it was emptied of patients to add to the widespread seeding of the community. Once dispersed, however, the epidemic again failed to maintain itself because of its low transmission efficiency and burnt itself out within two months without intervention.

Once again it is inconceivable that any hospital in a developed country could operate in the manner of the YMH so the possibility of a similar epidemic can be disregarded.

Other possible circumstances. While it is difficult to imagine that these special circumstances could recur with similar results in a developed country with a good health service, it is important to consider whether other circumstances peculiar to such countries might not increase the epidemic hazard. Two factors immediately come to mind. First, the medical care of the patients in both Sudan and Zaire was carried out with virtually no laboratory investigations. This eliminated one element of risk which would certainly be present in any modern hospital. It is a near certainty that a number of basic laboratory investigations ranging from bacteriological culture of stool, urine and blood through basic haematological tests to simple blood chemistry estimations would be ordered and probably carried out before a diagnosis of Ebola fever is seriously raised as a possibility. There is no practical way of preventing this. It must be accepted that it is not a human attribute to remain unflaggingly on the alert for something which never happens and the habit of including the possibility of Ebola or Lassa fevers in the differential diagnosis of Pyrexia of Unknown Origin (PUO) will inevitably lapse. Moreover, the onset of the infection is uncharacteristic being a progressive influenzal illness. Unless a history of a recent visit to the relevant part of Africa has been elicited at the outset, the physician may not be alerted to this possibility. On average, nurses in general hospital prick themselves with syringe needles between 10 and 30 times during the year and laboratory staff, particularly in haematology and biochemistry departments, are notoriously negligent in observing safety precautions when handling potentially infectious specimens. The incidence of hospital-acquired infections with hepatitis B gives ample evidence of this.

To this initial hazard must be added the requirement, after the true diagnosis has been made or suspected, for on-going laboratory monitoring of the factors required for clinical management. At this stage, there will be less danger of transferring the infection outside the hospital even if infection should occur in hospital staff members. Nevertheless a clear, if limited, hazard is present.

The second factor is that of mobility within the country. The type of person who will introduce infection will almost certainly be attuned to air travel and is likely to come from a stratum of society to which mobility is a way of life. While it may be too easy to over-rate this, in the Sudan and Zaire, where it would be much less formidable, infection reached Khartoum, 1,200 km to the north of Maridi, and Kinshasa, 1,000 km southwest of Yambuku – a total spread of 3,000 km.

Biology

The causative agent

Identity

The Marburg-Ebola group of viruses possess a morphology which distinguishes them from all other virus groups. They are highly pleomorphic RNA viruses which are synthesized in the cytoplasm of infected cells and mature by budding from the cell surface. They are thus covered with a lipoprotein outer membrane and are sensitive to inactivation by ether.

They are present in infected tissues and in tissue culture in three principal forms.

(1) Sinuous, cylindrical, membrane-covered particles of between 1 and 11 nm length and about 105 nm diameter. The outer, projection-bearing membrane covers an inner helix with a central core. There is an outer ether-soluble lipid envelope.[102] These sinuous forms tend to be conspicuously coiled and looped and may be branched. Loops may be open or closed, empty or filled with material arranged so as to suggest whorls of fused virus filaments.

(2) Separation of closed loops may give rise to ring forms resembling doughnuts of about 300–350 nm diameter. These are the dominant form in Marburg virus and were considered by Almeida *et al.*[57] to represent the mature form of the virus, but are less frequently seen in the case of Ebola virus.[110]

(3) Naked helices, presumably nucleocapsids of RNA-P material are seen devoid of outer membrane and are present in large arrays in the inclusion bodies.

This bizarre morphology is unique in the virus field. Although it has been suggested[123] that the virus should be classified with the rhabdoviruses, which include vesicular stomatitis virus and rabies virus, other authorities[101] maintain that the differences are too great to permit this grouping and suggest separate classification.

Stability and resistance

Little direct experimental information is available on the stability of Ebola virus but Simpson has summarized the more extensive knowledge regarding Marburg virus which closely resembles Ebola virus in physical properties as well as morphology and development.

The virus is inactivated by heating at 60°C for one hour but not at 56°C over the same period. It is stable when stored at −70°C, and even at room temperature shows little loss of infectivity for five weeks, but deteriorates thereafter to almost complete inactivation at eight weeks. Rapid inactivation occurs under ultra-violet irradiation.

As with other enveloped viruses it is inactivated by ether and sodium desoxycholate. Infectivity is destroyed by 1 per cent formaldehyde, 2 per cent sodium hypochlorite, 90 per cent acetone and 90 per cent methyl alcohol. It is also inactivated by 1 per cent Tego MGH and 2 per cent osmium tetroxide. The virus was not completely inactivated by 0.5 per cent phenol, 2 per cent cetrimide or 5 per cent trypsin.

From these results it may also be safely assumed that the virus is sensitive to gluteraldehyde.

There is no experimental evidence regarding the resistance of the virus to dessication or its survival in spilled blood, haemorrhagic excreta or vomitus, bloodstained fomites or contaminated dust on surfaces. However, its sensitivity to formalin, hypochlorite and, presumably, gluteraldehyde suggest that standard disinfection procedures should be effective.

Antigenic constitution and relationships

Marburg and Ebola viruses are antigenically distinct from each other[119, 128c] and from all other viruses against which they have been tested.[106] The European and South African strains of Marburg virus were antigenically identical, as are the Sudan and Zaire strains of the Ebola virus.

Mutability

There is no experimental evidence regarding the mutability of this virus group but Bowen[102, 105] has detected a difference in the lethality for both monkeys and guinea-pigs between the Sudan and Zaire strains, which is a much higher virulence.

Pathogenesis of infection

Portals of entry

The three outstanding mechanisms of transmission of infection have been by direct contact with infected blood, by transfer of gross contamination by attendant staff, and by inoculation either accidentally or through the use of contaminated, unsterilized instruments. In the community the close contact of nursing a sick patient has repeatedly been shown as necessary for transmission to occur, while persons living and sleeping in the same room, but without nursing contact, have not been infected. Apart from needle puncture, infection through skin abrasions, and by manual transfer of contamination to the mouth, nose or conjunctiva appear to be the most likely routes of infection. There is no evidence to suggest respiratory transmission.

Spread through the body

These viruses are highly invasive and there can be no doubt that generalization occurs by the haematogenous route.

Distribution and replication sites

As with all viruses which are generalized throughout the body with high concentrations in the blood, the identification of replication sites by virus titration of individual tissues is difficult. Bowen[102, 105] has quantitatively explored the distribution of Ebola virus in monkeys and guinea pigs and found high concentrations in the blood and in all the tissues examined. In both vervet and rhesus monkeys virus concentrations of about $10^{6.5}$/ml were found in the blood while the concentrations in the spleen, liver and lung were usually about one log higher. These findings parallel the demonstration of virus in liver, spleen and lung by electron microscopy. Replication probably also occurs in the adrenals and bone marrow and certainly in the testis.

Quantitative determinations are not available for Marburg virus but the extensive studies of the pathology of infection in monkeys and guinea pigs carried out by Simpson and his colleagues[102, 132] indicate a very similar distribution of both macroscopic and microscopic lesions which correspond closely to the findings in man.[123]

Shedding from the body

The most important shedding of virus from the body occurs through haemorrhage. The haemorrhagic diathesis may develop as early as the third day, as evidenced by the presence of melaena, but major haemorrhages do not usually occur before the second week when, in severe cases, bleeding may occur from any body orifice. When diarrhoea and vomiting occur this may lead to gross environmental contamination with highly infective material. Shedding of virus by other means appears to be minimal. There does not seem to be a true pharyngitis although severe dryness of the mouth and throat is present in many patients[128b] and there is frequently a dry cough with severe chest pain. The demonstration of virus replication in the lung of monkeys[105, 109] would indicate a risk of respiratory transmission but this occurs rarely if at all and Peters *et al.* had little success in isolating virus from throat washings.[123] These findings show that it may be that the infectious period of the patient closely parallels the haemorrhagic phase of the disease and the degree of haemorrhage will determine the degree of danger from any patient. Patients who do not develop a haemorrhagic tendency will be relatively non-infective.

Clinical factors

It is clear from the clinical nature of the disease that general supportive measures with control of dehydration and haemorrhage are critically important in therapy and may demand close laboratory monitoring. The high virus concentrations in the blood could make such monitoring very hazardous and demands extreme care in the taking, handling, transportation and testing of specimens.

Besides general clinical management, specific treatment must depend upon the availability of convalescent serum or plasma. The benefits of such treatment have not been formally proven but results indicate its effectiveness. Certainly the combination of immune plasma and interferon therapy given to Mr Platt, who suffered a laboratory infection at Porton, appeared to effect an immediate control of his viraemia. A similar result was obtained in treating an experimental infection in a rhesus monkey.[102] The value of interferon cannot at this time be assessed. In Platt's case it was given along with immune plasma and the separate effects could not be judged. Bowen[102] tested the effects of interferon in experimental infections in monkeys using the Zaire strain of virus and obtained results suggesting that there was a slight prolongation of survival time even though the animals died.

Prophylaxis

With regard to prophylaxis, no vaccine is yet available. The potential value of vaccine therapy has, however, been shown by Bowen.[58] On day 56 after infection, he challenged the rhesus monkey, whose infection had been controlled by immune plasma therapy, using the Sudan strain of Ebola virus. The monkey showed no clinical signs of illness and developed neither fever or viraemia. On day 81, it was rechallenged with the more virulent Zaire strain at a dosage of 10^4 guinea pig infectious units – a dose which would be expected to be uniformly fatal. The monkey developed a slight fever and went off its food between days 4–6 and viraemia to a level of 10^1 IU/ml occurred for three days. There was no other sign of illness. While too much dependence cannot be placed upon this isolated result, it does suggest that convalescent immunity can be solid and prophylactic vaccination might be effective.

9

Plague

Epidemiology

1. History and analysis

The ancient origins of plague are shrouded in mythology and historians still do not agree on the interpretation of accounts of epidemics occurring in the pre-Christian era. Whatever its origins, there is no doubt that plague has been one of the most devastating epidemic diseases to afflict mankind. According to Topley and Wilson,[148] during the 1,500 years following the birth of Christ, there are records of 109 epidemics including the great plague of Justinian and the Black Death of the fourteenth century. From 1500 to 1720, there were 45 pandemics. Two centuries of comparative quiescence followed although there were major epidemics in Marseilles, Moscow, the Balkans and Egypt. At the beginning of this century, the main impact of the disease was in India where between 1898 and 1918 more than 10 million deaths were recorded in a series of annual epidemics centred on Bombay. During this same period, and as late as 1921, major epidemics occurred in Manchuria, Mongolia and China.

The disease was introduced to Glasgow, Sydney and San Francisco in 1900. The last of these introductions has had serious long-term consequences since the infection escaped into the indigenous rodent population and is now established as a sylvatic zoonosis throughout the western third of the country. Its eastward spread continues and appears to be at the rate of one meridian every 10 years. The number of human cases which occur annually is small and recorded cases in the US have remained below 20 per year. The US is now one of only three major natural foci of the disease in the world, the other two are South Africa and Northern China. This is why plague must be considered.

Today the disease is primarily sylvatic, involving over 200 different species of rodents, and affects man only as an accidental infection. In this form it is not an epidemic threat and it becomes so only when it spreads to those populations of *Rattus rattus*, the black rat, which are in close contact with human populations. Although the animal associations of *Yersinia pestis*, the plague bacillus, are extremely complex and variable across the world, the association of human epidemic spread with the black rat and its flea, *Xenopsylla cheopsis*, appears to be universal.

This association was first established in 1905 by the English Plague Commission in India[148] whose classical studies also established the complex cycle where human epidemic plague was maintained as a seasonal event. This was shown to be a threefold cycle originating with the brown sewer rat, *Rattus norvegicus*, which was the basic reservoir of disease in India at that time. Each year an exacerbation of the enzootic state began at the end of December and rapidly reached epizootic proportions, peaking in February. This event was followed about 10 days later by a similar epizootic among the domesticated black rats, peaking in March. This in turn, was followed by the human epidemic, peaking in March and April.

Human plague was shown to be transmitted by the rat flea from *Rattus rattus* to man and the severity of the epidemic depended on the density of the rat population and the closeness of its association with the human population. Direct transmission from person to person is extremely rare and even at the time of the Black Death it was noted that those visiting the sick were at no greater risk of developing the disease than those who did not.

Clinical types of plague

The clinical type of disease in these epidemics was the classical bubonic plague characterized by the development of intensely painful abscesses or buboes in the regional lymph nodes, usually the groin, draining the site of the infected flea-bite.

There is an incubation period of two to six days followed by a rapid progression of the illness, development of septicaemia and death sometimes occurs within hours. The case-fatality rate is in excess of 60 per cent.

Some cases develop a fulminating septicaemia with such rapidity that death occurs before buboes have time to develop and in this 'septicaemic' form of the disease, the case-fatality rate is 100 per cent.

Today in Western communities, bubonic plague, including its clinical extension of septicaemic plague, does not represent an epidemic threat since there is no critical close domestic association between the black rat and man. In the absence of a potential for person-to-person spread, no community epidemic could develop. This limitation, however, does not hold for the third clinical variety of the disease – pneumonic plague.

Pneumonic involvement is an inevitable accompaniment of the septicaemia which occurs as the terminal event in the bubonic form, but pneumonia is a secondary development, does not usually dominate the clinical picture, and is clinically apparent only in some 5 per cent of cases. Occasionally, the situation is reversed and pneumonia becomes the dominating feature of the illness. Such cases may then be highly infectious in their own right by direct respiratory person-to-person spread and may initiate a community epidemic which no longer requires the presence of the rat and the rat flea. Crowding and mobility in modern communities provides potential for rapid and uncontrollable spread of such a respiratory infection. This is well illustrated by the behaviour of the epidemic, and even more so by pandemic influenza. Since pneumonic plague has a case-fatality rate approaching 100 per cent, an outbreak in an urban community could be truly devastating.

The factors which govern such a change in the behaviour are unclear. More is required than just the development of cases of plague pneumonia which are not rare among the sporadic cases which occur annually in the endemic areas. In north China and Manchuria, bubonic plague was, at the beginning of this century, a summer event while the pneumonic form caused winter epidemics. This appeared to be caused by gross overcrowding in insanitary conditions in high humidity – conditions which are not likely in most developed communities. The route of invasion of the body by the causative organism is also of importance. For a primary pneumonia to develop, the infective dose must reach the lung and establish itself there, otherwise the pneumonia will remain a secondary feature as in the classical bubonic form of the disease and the potential for person-to-person spread may be lost. Lung penetration, however, demands a small particle size aerosol with a mean particle diameter of less than 5 μm. Such particles are usually produced in very small proportion from cases of lung infection in which the infective agent is embedded in mucus secretions which tend to dry to large diameter particles. The effect has been clearly shown in the laboratory in plague-infected guinea-pigs.[115] Animals exposed by the respiratory route to 1 μm particles develop a primary pneumonia and are infectious to control animals caged with them. The infected control animals, however, do not develop a primary pneumonia but succumb to the lymphatic type of disease which follows invasion via the upper respiratory tract and is analogous to bubonic plague in man. Such animals do not pass on the infection to controls caged with them and it is not possible to initiate a continued epidemic by the respiratory route.

Climate also appears to be critically important in the epidemiology of plague with temperature and humidity the principal factors. In India, their influence was not primarily upon the organism and its transmissibility, but upon the animal reservoirs and the flea vector.

The complexity of the factors governing the epidemiology of plague make it difficult to assess the danger of a community outbreak of pneumonic plague following the chance introduction of a case of plague pneumonia into a susceptible urban community. No community outbreak has occurred during the 80 years when the agent has been loose in the US. This suggests that the risk is not great; the WHO Expert Committee has stated that: 'There is no longer a danger of extensive pandemics or epidemics of plague except in the event of war or other calamities'.[152]

2. Case-fatality rate

In the absence of antibacterial treatment, the case-fatality rate in plague is high, about 60 per cent in the bubonic form and approaching 100 per cent in the septicaemic and pneumonic forms. With early diagnosis and prompt antibacterial therapy, the fatality rate may be reduced to below 20 per cent.

3. Community and seasonal incidence

No generalization can be made about these two factors since they vary with the country and locale. In India, the community incidence during the epidemic exacerbatioñ was high and the epizootics and subsequent epidemics occurred during the cooler weather. By contrast, the epidemics of bubonic plague in northern China occurred during the summer and tended to alternate with the pneumonic form during the winter. In the US, the sporadic cases of plague which occur each year fall predominantly in summer when the chances of contact with small rodents are greatest.

4. Ecology

The ecology of the sylvatic plague varies throughout the world and is too complex for detailed treatment here. A very wide range of animals is susceptible to the disease and a wide range of vectors including various species of fleas, lice and ticks are involved in transmission.

The principal animal reservoirs are small rodents which do not normally associate closely with man, but human infections and small outbreaks affecting farmsteads may occur if infection spreads to the very susceptible black rat. In South Africa an important reservoir is *Mastomys natalensis* which, in North West Africa and Mozambique, is the principal known reservoir of Lassa fever.

5. Vector requirements

Arthropod vectors are an essential requirement for transmitting sylvatic plague among rodents and many biting ectoparasites including fleas; lice and ticks may also be involved. Epizootic transmission in rat populations is flea-borne and human involvement depends largely upon the biting specificity of the fleas involved. It is the catholic taste of the rat fleas *Xenopsylla cheopsis* and *Nosopsyllus fasciatus*, together with the domesticated habits of the black rat which make this combination so dangerous to man in rat-infested communities.

By comparison, human fleas are poor transmitters of plague. Therefore the scarcity of man-flea-man transmission and the dependence of human epidemic bubonic plague upon rat-flea-man transmission is based upon a concurrent rat plague epizootic.

6. Mechanisms of transmission of infection

Transmission of infection among the many animal species involved in the maintenance of sylvatic plague depends primarily upon the biting activity of ectoparasites. Carnivores may also become infected, presumably by eating the infected rodents which form the main reservoir. Hunters may also contract infection through blood contamination from infected carcasses. Sporadic infection in man is in fact very similar to the pattern found with Tularaemia. Transmission within the rat population and from rat to man is almost exclusively dependent upon the rat fleas *Xenopsylla cheopsis* and *Nosopsyllus fasciatus*.

Person-to-person transmission of bubonic plague in man is unusual but infection may occur from handling infected dressings or linen contaminated by contaminated discharges, especially from ruptured lymphatic abscesses or buboes.

Direct person-to-person transmission does, however, occur in pneumonic plague and is by the respiratory route.

7. Infectious period of the patient

Patients do not become infectious until after the onset of clinical illness and then only if infected discharges are shed from the body or if pneumonic symptoms with a cough develop. The disease is primarily a septicaemia with internal abscess formation in many organs but without external shedding.

Under antibacterial treatment patients who respond become rapidly non-infective and Poland[149] recommends strict isolation for 48 hours after commencement of specific therapy in all cases as a precaution if pneumonic involvement has occurred, but continuing isolation only if respiratory symptoms or purulent discharges are present. If not, isolation may be lifted.

8. Transmissibility

Person-to-person transmissibility in plague is virtually restricted to the pneumonic form of the disease except under conditions of very close nursing contact when purulent exudates or discharges constitute a hazard. The true degree of transmissibility of the pneumonic disease is, however, very difficult to assess. In secondary pneumonia, which occurs in 5 per cent of bubonic cases and is marked by cough and bloody sputum, there is a clear danger of transmission, but Poland[149] points out that:

> Respiratory spread occurs primarily to persons in close and prolonged contact with the case. Hence, secondary cases have occurred most frequently in medical personnel or household contacts who are directly involved with the care of the patient and infrequently in household contacts (children and other adults) not intimately associated with the patient.

He also states that since 1925 no spread to contacts has been detected in the US. In view of the constant annual trickle of cases, this is a significant observation.

In primary pneumonic plague, the situation is different, probably because of the very much higher concentration of organisms in the lungs which are expelled by coughing. Through its devastating epidemics and high mortality in Manchuria and northern China early in the century and has become known as one of the most infectious diseases known to man with a transmissibility comparable to that of influenza. Whether this reputation is fully justified, however, seems doubtful. These epidemics have all occurred under conditions of gross overcrowding where people were huddled together in hot, humid, unventilated insanitary conditions designed to keep out the bitter northern Asiatic winter. The conditions where limited outbreaks occurred in India were scarcely more comparable to those of developed communities today. Few particles derived from coughing are small enough to penetrate the lungs, so high concentrations of aerosolized organisms must be generated to ensure primary pneumonic invasion. This is a requirement for this form of the disease since upper respiratory invasion would lead to primary lymphatic spread to which pulmonary involvement, if it occurred, would be secondary as in bubonic plague. This requirement is in marked contrast to influenzal transmission where the primary focus of infection is in the naso-pharynx where the majority of particles derived from coughing and sneezing will lodge.

Clearly, the patient with pneumonic plague would be very dangerous in crowded public transport or other gathering places and could infect numerous secondary cases. It is less certain whether an epidemic chain-reaction could be set up even in a crowded urban community. Moreover, the clinical nature of the disease would tend to limit transmission since the onset is abrupt and progresses rapidly with death occurring in untreated cases within hours or a few days. Cases would, therefore, be ambulatory for only a short period.

As with Lassa and Ebola-Marburg fevers, it would seem that the main danger would be to health care staff and special precautions to protect against respiratory exposure would be required.

Biology

The causitive organism

Identity

Yersinia pestis is a small ovoid gram-negative bacillus showing conspicuous bipolar 'safety-pin' staining in smears derived from infected organs or pus. Its natural habitat is in animals, primarily rodents, and is capable of infecting a wide range of animals including man.

In vivo, the bacillus develops a conspicuous capsule which renders it resistant to phagocytosis. *In vitro*, it grows slowly on nutrient solid media at 37°C giving pin-point colonies after overnight incubation. Optimal growth temperature range is 27–30°C.

Stability and resistance

The organism is not especially resistant. It can be killed at a temperature of 55°C in 15 minutes and can be rapidly inactivated by standard disinfectants. It survives for only a few days at room temperature in dried pus or discharges.

Antigenic constitution

The antigenic constitution is complex but only one antigenic type exists. A capsular virulence antigen is formed but for full virulence, three other non-capsular antigens are required. Fully virulent organisms derived from the body are markedly inhibitory to phagocytosis unless treated with anti-capsular antibody. Some antigenic components are shared with *Y. pseudotuberculosis*.

Mutability

Research has suggested that the organism has a limited capacity for variation in virulence in nature. It develops enhanced virulence during rapid passage in the early stages of a growing epizootic and then relapses into a less virulent stage permitting the development of indolent lesions and latency in the rat at the end of the epizootic period. Under laboratory conditions, avirulent strains and strains of low virulence can be identified.

Pathogenesis of infection

Portals of entry

The portal of entry of the organism in bubonic plague is transdermal by direct inoculation following the bite of an infected flea. Fleas become infected by taking a blood meal from a plague-stricken rat and the organism multiplies in the rat blood held in the proventriculus of the flea which leaves the corpse of the rat and transfers to a new host, which may be a human. Multiplication of the bacteria may completely block the proventriculus and prevent access of blood to the stomach and such a 'blocked' flea becomes intensely hungry. Its vigorous attempts to feed break up the bacterial mass in its proventriculus and forcibly regurgitate blood and bacteria into the tissues of the new host.

In man the flea-bite is frequently on the lower leg where a small focal lesion may develop. Lymphatic spread then leads to abscess formation in the regional lymph nodes with the development of the classical buboes. This stage is followed by haematogenous generalization and development of necrotic abscesses which may involve any organ. Pneumonia develops in about 5 per cent of the cases.

In pneumonic plague, the portal of entry is the lung alveoli following inhalation of organisms, which rapidly spread to the blood.through direct penetration to the alveolar capillaries.

Replication sites

The organism is capable of multiplying and producing lesions in any organ of the body. In bubonic plague the sequence is: focal multiplication at the site of flea-bite, multiplication in the regional lymph-nodes to form buboes, and generalization with abscess formation in many organs. Plague is one of the few diseases where active multiplication also occurs in the blood.

In the pneumonic form the primary replication site is the lung alveoli and death usually follows so quickly that there is little time for the remote lesions to develop.

Spread through the body

In the bubonic form of plague, the initial spread is lymphatic followed by blood invasion and haematogenous dispersal through the body. In the pneumonic form, the lymphatics are not involved; the blood is reached directly by alveolar penetration so that septicaemia with haematogenous dispersal is very rapid.

Distribution

Following onset of septicaemia the organism is distributed throughout the entire body.

Shedding from the body

In the purely bubonic form of plague, the organism is shed from the body only as a result of external rupture of an abscess or by haemorrhage of infected blood.

In the pneumonic form, shedding also occurs by the respiratory tract with the generation of dangerous aerosols derived from the coughing of bloodstained secretions teeming with plague bacilli.

Tracheostomies on pneumonic patients are especially dangerous, as is handling dressings and other objects contaminated with pus or blood.

Clinical factors

Therapy and prophylaxis.[149] *Yersinia pestis* is very susceptible to the actions of sulphonamides, streptomycin, tetracyclines and chloramphenicol. Streptomycin is most often used for therapy and sulfadiazine or trisulfapyrimidines for prophylaxis. Penicillins are not effective.

Treatment must be started early to be effective and all contacts should be given prophylactic sulfonamides. Nonspecific supportive therapy may be required to control shock, high fever, convulsions and diffuse intravascular coagulation. A heat-killed vaccine prepared from *Y. pestis* is available.

Section Three

Response

10

Summary of Present Situation

The emergence of apparently new and highly dangerous diseases during the past 10 years has compelled Western countries to face the necessity for developing special measures to prevent their introduction into urbanized communities with the ensuing danger of uncontrollable epidemic spread. The two diseases which have caused this reaction are Lassa and Ebola-Marburg fevers, but there is also the serious threat from other haemorrhagic fevers and the ancient pestilences of cholera and plague.

The preliminary examination in Section I led to the conclusion that, today only smallpox, yellow fever, Lassa fever, Ebola-Marburg fever and plague constitute a sufficient epidemic threat to developed communities to need detailed study. The examination of these diseases in Section II suggests the following summary conclusions.

Smallpox

Smallpox is the oldest known viral haemorrhagic fever. It is the only one exclusive to man and the only one spread by the respiratory route. Although it is less readily transmissible than might be expected from its route of transmission, it spreads rapidly and extensively in susceptible communities and, because the virus is resistant to inactivation by drying, it presents major problems in control and containment.

The disease has now been declared 'eradicated' from the world and no longer demands special public health precautions. It should not be forgotten, that closely related viruses exist in unidentified animal reservoirs and the possibility of its use as a biological weapon cannot be confidently dismissed.

Yellow fever

Yellow fever is ineradicably established in the monkey populations of western and central Africa and northern South America. Trinidad is the only Caribbean island where the disease is now known to be endemic. In endemic areas, outbreaks of sylvan yellow fever are not uncommon and occasional major epidemics, such as the one in Nigeria in 1969–70, may occur in the human population.

The epidemic threat outside the endemic areas lies in the wide distribution of the vector mosquito, *Aedes aegypti*, in the two major receptive areas of the world – the Caribbean and southeastern Asia. In both these areas the dengue virus, transmitted by this same vector, has produced widespread epidemics in recent years showing that the potential for spread of urban yellow fever is present. In addition, the susceptibility to infection of the rhesus monkey of India and southeastern Asia suggests a dangerous possibility of establishing a permanent sylvatic reservoir if the virus is introduced.

Since direct person-to-person transmission does not occur, the epidemic potential of the disease in man is strictly limited to the tropical and sub-tropical distribution of the *Aedes aegypti* mosquito. The Theiler vaccine provides solid immunity.

Lassa fever

Lassa fever is a zoonosis with a wide endemic distribution in northwest Africa, and rodent carriage of the causative virus, or at least of a closely related strain, has recently been demonstrated in Mozambique without human infection. The only known reservoir of the virus is the multimammate rat *Mastomys natalensis*, which is distributed throughout Africa and far exceeds the known distribution of Lassa fever. Transmission of infection from rodents to man is probably by urinary or faecal contamination of the human environment. Arthropod vectors are not thought to be involved.

The incubation period of the human disease is usually 6–14 days. The longest incubation period on record is 17 days. The early clinical picture is that of a non-specific influenzal illness of progressive severity passing, after about the sixth day, into the more characteristic pattern of severe ulcerative pharyngitis, diarrhoea, vomiting and haemorrhagic diathesis. Death, when it occurs, is usually around day 12–14 of illness. The case-fatality rate in hospitalized patients is about 20–30 per cent. Many mild and sub-clinical infections, however, occur in the community and the infection-fatality rate is less than 5 per cent.

Most community infections are acquired from the rodent reservoir. Person-to-person infection is infrequent. In hospital, however, person-to-person spread is a dangerous source of nosocomial infections among medical and nursing staff caring for Lassa patients. Infection may also be transferred to other patients and the danger to both patients and staff is greatly enhanced when nursing techniques are inadequate. Transmission requires close contact with a patient during the height of his illness and is mediated by direct contamination with infectious body fluids or effluvia. Virus is usually present in pharyngeal secretions from onset but, despite an almost constant cough, respiratory transmission rarely occurs. Persistent viruria may develop but has not been incriminated in transfer of infection. Many nosocomial infections have been due to parenteral inoculation of the virus as a result of syringe-needle or autopsy accident.

Person-to-person transmissibility is so low that, in the absence of the rodent reservoir, the disease in its present form is devoid of epidemic potential in the community. This situation could be dangerously altered if the virus mutates towards pneumotropism or acquires the ability to multiply to high concentration in the oropharynx.

Ebola-Marburg fever

Ebola and Marburg virus infections may be regarded as a single entity of variable lethality, although the causative viruses differ antigenically. The disease is probably a zoonosis although no animal reservoir has yet been identified and only serological evidence exists for its endemic incidence in man. Arthropod transmission may be involved since the virus can multiply in the mosquito *Aedes aegypti* under laboratory conditions. Direct person-to-person transmission only occurs under conditions of the closest physical contact or by iatrogenic means, when the direct inoculation of virus-contaminated medications has proved to be the most dangerous. The incubation period is usually 6–8 days but may be shorter following direct inoculation and, in one instance of contact transmission, may have been as long as 21 days.

The early clinical picture is non-specific until the progressive development of severe prostration, headache, muscle and abdominal pain, vomiting, diarrhoea and haemorrhagic diathesis establish the characteristic clinical pattern from about the sixth day. The mouth and throat are extremely dry, but there is no true pharyngitis. Respiratory involvement is variable. The case-fatality rate was 23 per cent in the European outbreak, 53 per cent in Sudan and 88 per cent in Zaire.

Transmissibility is of a very low order and the disease could not sustain itself, even in a fully susceptible community living under primitive, overcrowded conditions. Each of the three epidemic episodes was due to locally prevailing special circumstances. Under Western conditions, the disease would have little epidemic potential in the community.

Some evidence exists to suggest mutability in the virus and it is possible that the Zaire strain is a derivative of the Sudan strain with enhanced virulence.

Plague

The basic pattern of human plague is that of a zoonosis dependent on the close association of the principal rodent reservoir, *Rattus rattus*, the black rat, with man. When the rat population is large and the association close, epizootic spread among the rats is reflected in epidemic spread in the human population. Under these conditions, transfer of infection is from rodent to man and is mediated by the bite of the rat flea, *Xenopsylla cheopis*. Deposition of the causative organism into the tissues and blood in this manner gives rise to a spreading lymphatic and septicaemic infection which manifests itself in the 'bubonic' form of the disease.

After an incubation period of about two to five days, rapid development of illness follows, marked by extreme prostration and the development of the characteristic lymphatic abscesses or 'buboes'. These are hard in the initial stages but later become fluctuant and may rupture to discharge a copious foul-smelling pus teeming with plague bacilli. The case-fatality rate is usually above 60 per cent in the bubonic form, but the disease may also take a fulminant septicaemic course with a uniformly fatal outcome, death occurring within hours after onset. Person-to-person transfer of infection in the bubonic and septicaemic forms of the disease is rare.

By contrast, the pneumonic form of plague is primarily a respiratory infection where transmission occurs from person-to-person directly by the respiratory route without the intervention of the rat. The transmission rate is high and epidemic spread is no longer limited by the speed of travel of plague-infected rats so that major epidemics can develop very rapidly with a clinical picture of a fulminating pneumonia and a case-fatality rate approaching 100 per cent. The factors governing the switch from the bubonic to the pneumonic form of the disease are not known, nor is it known whether all plague pneumonias have the potential for initiating a pneumonic epidemic. This seems unlikely.

Pneumonia is not uncommon in sporadic plague infections[146, 147] although the majority are the bubonic form, but epidemic transmission is rare and appears to be very sensitive to environmental conditions requiring especially high humidity and gross overcrowding. Experiments suggest that in guinea pigs, although animals which developed pneumonia following exposure to plague by the respiratory route with 1 μm particles are infectious to control animals caged with them, the second generation of infection leads to upper respiratory invasion by the organism with *lymphatic spread* instead of *pneumonic involvement*. Animals with this type of disease, which corresponds to the bubonic form, are not infectious even by close contact. It therefore seems unlikely that there is a serious threat of epidemic pneumonic plague in developed communities despite the wide distribution of the causative organism in South

Africa, US and Vietnam. These three areas, together with the southern USSR and northern China now form the major wild plague foci in the world and expert opinion considers that 'there is no longer a danger of extensive pandemics or epidemics of plague except in the event of war or other calamities'.[152] Even in the endemic areas, the incidence of human plague appears to be small and, in the US, has not risen above 20 cases per year during the last 10 years. It may be concluded that the threat from this disease is more theoretical.

Future possibilities

The remaining diseases examined in Section One are either lacking in epidemic potential or are wholly dependent upon their rodent reservoirs or arthropod vectors and so are strictly limited in their geographical distribution. Allowance must be made, however, for two further possibilities.

First, it may be confidently expected that in the future, new diseases will emerge as human infections. They may have been present but unrecognized in local populations as Lassa fever was in West Africa, or they may be zoonoses which have not previously been encountered by man, or at least have not invaded the human population with sufficient emphasis to be recognized as individual entities. There is no way to forecast the results of new contacts of this type. They may indeed result in epidemics of high lethality as in Zaire or the animal disease may prove to be entirely non-transmissible to man as was presumably the case with Simian haemorrhagic fever which since 1964 has caused lethal epidemics in monkeys in Russia, the US and Britain without a single case of human infection.[141-3]

Although the future emergence of 'new' diseases may be expected to occur from time to time, it seems unlikely that any lethal disease of high epidemic potential could still be lurking in some unpenetrated corner of the world awaiting the arrival of man for its uncontrollable release into the human community. It is far more probable that any newly emergent disease, however virulent, will have the same low degree of transmissibility as Lassa and Ebola fevers.

The second factor, which could well be of greater concern, is that of mutability in the haemorrhagic fever viruses known today. In the absence of flying insect vector transmission, the epidemic potential of the known diseases is intimately related to their potential for respiratory transmission. In both Lassa and Ebola fevers, this potential is low to the extent that neither disease could maintain itself as a community epidemic without the special factors already described. On the other hand, there is frequently pneumonic involvement with virus replication in the lung in both diseases. In Lassa fever, virus is also present in the pharynx and severe pharyngitis and cough are constant features of the disease. In the Jos episode of 1970, the index case was admitted as a case of pneumonia and thought to have initiated an outbreak of aerosol-spread infection.[51]

The danger lies in the fact that enhancement of virulence and pneumotropism by passage has been repeatedly demonstrated in the laboratory. This is particularly the case with influenza virus and it was certainly a pneumotropic variant of high virulence which caused the 1918–19 influenza pandemic and killed an estimated 20 million people despite a case-fatality rate of only 3 per cent. In influenza virus, high transmissibility is already present, and pneumotropism and high virulence are linked properties. In Lassa and Ebola fevers, virulence is already high even in the absence of marked pneumotropism; only communicability is lacking. If it is true that the infectiousness of individual patients is related to the level of virus in their pharyngeal secretions, a relatively trivial adaptation towards enhanced replication in the respiratory tract could transform either virus into a devastatingly dangerous threat.

Today, there is little evidence regarding mutability of these viruses, but there is evidence to suggest that their behaviour is not uniform across the African continent. Lassa fever, for instance, is endemic in the human population of northwest Africa but no human cases have been identified in Mozambique[98] despite the presence of the virus among the rodent population. In the case of Ebola fever there was a striking difference in lethality between the epidemics in Sudan and Zaire. Preliminary experiments at Porton suggest that there is a corresponding difference in virulence for laboratory animals between the strains of virus isolated from the two localities. The Zaire strain has also exhibited passage adaptability to guinea pigs in the laboratory, with increasing lethality and shortening the time to death.

If these findings are confirmed, the implications could be serious. Although it has not been possible to establish a positive link between the two epidemics, it is known that there was frequent traffic between the two areas involved and it seems very likely that the Zaire outbreak was derived from the one in the Sudan. If so, the confirmation of a markedly enhanced virulence in the derived Zaire strain of virus would be evidence of a disquieting mutability in the genome of the Ebola virus. Even more disquieting is van der Groen and Pattyn's suggestion that the strains of Ebola virus responsible for the Sudan and Zaire outbreaks arose from a presumably avirulent virus endemic in northwestern Zaire, well outside the observed epidemic areas. The suggestion of avirulence is implicit in the relatively high incidence of seropositivity which they measured[139] in the absence of any observed disease, since it is inconceivable that this could have occurred with a virus as lethal as that which caused the 1976 epidemics.

11

Control and Containment

From the facts summarized in this discussion, and from a conservative extrapolation of them it is possible to construct a reasonable pattern of response to the possible inadvertent introduction of any of the designated diseases into a susceptible Western community.

Table 11 summarizes the situation.

TABLE 11   Summary of diseases

1	Smallpox
2	Yellow fever
3	Plague
4	Lassa fever
5	Ebola-Marburg fever

Epidemic threat

(1) Smallpox has been eradicated and is controllable by established procedures.
(2) Yellow fever constitutes a threat only in the geographical distribution of its mosquito vectors. Urban yellow fever can be controlled by reducing the population of *Aedes aegypti* and by immunization.
(3) Plagues at present poses only a theoretical threat.
(4, 5) Lassa Fever and Ebola-Marburg fever pose little epidemic threat to the community.

Hazard to staff

The danger to hospital staff from any of these diseases is formidable and special measures are required for their protection.

Containment

(1) Containing smallpox demands special measures and facilities beyond the present capacity of general hospitals.

(2) Lassa and Ebola-Marburg fevers have so far shown minimal person-to-person transmissibility and standard isolation procedures practiced in general hospitals should effectively contain them. This also seems to be true of plague.

(3) Containment of yellow fever demands efficient anti-mosquito precautions.

The theory and practice of control and containment may be considered within this framework, and it should be appreciated that the interests of public health and of the patient may conflict.

Theory and practice

Objectives

The objectives for procedures to control and contain an infectious disease are: to prevent spread of the disease in the population at risk; to protect personnel involved in the care of cases of the disease or in the handling of infectious materials; and to contain the infectious agent within a defined locality. The requirements will vary not only with the characteristics of the particular disease but also with the environment in which they are intended to operate.

In the present context, the community and hospital environments will be considered separately.

The purpose of this analysis is to examine the situations in which procedures must operate, the precise nature of the threat which they must be designed to meet and to identify an appropriate scale of response. The requirements will clearly differ according to the degree of infectivity and mode of transmission of the individual diseases. Their complexity and stringency will also vary with the degree of safety to be achieved. It ultimately becomes the task of the responsible health authorities to select an appropriate scale of response, based upon an informed assessment of risk and practicable financial outlay.

This section will define the alternative techniques and procedures available for control and containment and discuss their relative merits regarding safety and patient management.

Control and containment in the community

Control and containment in the community is primarily a matter of swift and effective public health response. It entails the following sequence of definable elements.

1. **Identification.** Identification is a complex process in an isolated case. All the threatening diseases require laboratory tests for their positive identification and these may take a week or even longer to complete. Action must be taken on a suspicion and astute assessment by the diagnosing physician is required. A high index of suspicion must be balanced by caution based upon awareness of risk considering the occupation and recent movements of the patient and the detailed distribution of the suspected disease.

Emond,[165] the leading authority in this field, has suggested a logical classification of Lassa fever suspects which may be used to guide decisions regarding precautionary behaviour. The difficulty of their application is evident from the fact that about the same proportion of patients from each of his categories were actually placed under full isolation. Clearly, only clinical judgement, based upon experience, can be relied upon at this stage, so provision must be made for prompt availability of specialist consultation. Even so, a truly informed judgement is likely to be difficult to obtain in most Western countries.

2. **Segregation.** When suspicion is aroused, immediate action must be taken to segregate the patient and this will depend upon the location of the patient and the facilities immediately available. Suspect patients may be first encountered in any one of four probable sets of circumstances.

(a) *In the community*
   1. A place of residence might be a family home where segregation from the community would usually be simple,

although the family members would be liable to exposure, or it might be a public residence such as a hotel which could raise many additional problems. In either case, an urgent decision must be made as to whether the patient should be hospitalized immediately or whether a firm diagnosis should be made first or at least a preliminary observation period be maintained. The nature of the disease suspected would markedly affect this decision. If a patient were suspected of smallpox, a short delay for electron-microscopic examination of vesicle fluid would possibly be justified but prolonged delay before establishing institutional isolation would not. Similarly, suspected pneumonic plague would demand immediate isolation in hospital, although precipitate action would not be so urgent in a PUO from West Africa.

The type of action would also be governed by the availability and accessibility of adequate isolation facilities. This could be an especially important factor in North America where hospitals have the right to refuse patients, particularly in the US where the great majority of hospitals are privately owned, profit-making institutions.

2. A physician's office or consulting room would present different problems since segregation could probably not be effected *in situ* and it is likely that few physicians have prepared contingency plans for such an eventuality. The choice would lie between the patient's home and hospital admission, either choice raising the immediate problems of transportation and disinfection of the physician's own premises. Again, action will be markedly influenced by the nature of the disease suspected.

3. In hospital, the precise action might vary according to the sophistication of the hospital, whether or not the patient had already been admitted, and the availability of another special isolation facility.

The immediate action required is the most effective segregation of the patient and in most instances this will require an *ad hoc* improvisation which will usually fall short of the desirable.

The remaining types of first encounter are likely to be

much less frequent, leave fewer options, and have been subjected to examination and contingency planning – although if there are no designated isolation facilities, this is not necessarily very effective. Most international ports of entry have medical facilities where patients can be segregated and the main problems would be hospital acceptance and transportation.

(b) *Port of entry*

It is highly unlikely that an infected individual whose condition has not been recognized by the crew of the carrier during the journey will be intercepted at the port of entry. Only one instance of interception is on record and that was accidental. A passenger, returning to Toronto, was so ill that she fell in the airport after arrival, giving herself a scalp-wound which required suturing. She was taken as a stretcher case to the nearest general hospital where the minor surgery was carried out and it was only then that her general condition was appreciated. She spent the next nine days in the intensive care unit being treated for pneumonia before Lassa fever was suspected. The suspicion was never in fact confirmed.

By contrast, in 1961, there were five introductions into the UK of smallpox from Pakistan where the disease was known to be epidemic and one of the cases even vomited on the apron after disembarking; yet even this case was not intercepted at the port of entry.

(c) *En route via aircraft or ship*

In the days when most passenger travel was by ship there was every possibility that incubating diseases would show themselves before the ships arrived at their destinations, so all major passenger ships carried doctors who were experienced in the diseases they might encounter. The principal hazard at that time was from smallpox and the journey from the Asian endemo-epidemic areas to the susceptible Western communities was long enough to act as an efficient quarantine period. The length of a journey from India to Britain was such that exanthemata usually declared themselves before the ships reached Malta. Specimens from suspicious cases could be flown to London and examined by the Central Public Health Laboratory in time for a positive or negative diagnosis to await the ship's arrival three days later.

Unfortunately, these days are past and sea-borne traffic is now only marginally relevant by comparison with the volume of air travel. Air passengers are not subject to medical scrutiny, and anxiety and air-sickness are so common among travellers they they might disguise the symptoms and signs of more serious illness. The likelihood of a passenger with VHF being detected en route, especially if he wished to conceal his illness, is probably even less than the chances of detection after arrival and disembarkation. There is no record of any major infectious disease being detected by the crew of an aircraft so that warning could be radioed ahead to the port of entry.

(d) *Dedicated aero-medical evacuation*

It may be assumed that dedicated aero-medical evacuation of a suspected haemorrhagic fever case would not be undertaken without an advance, complete plan for transport and hospitalization after the patient's arrival at his destination.

3. **Notification.** Notification is the necessary preliminary for setting into motion the measures which together constitute the public health response. These should be governed by contingency planning with respect to 4, 5 and 6.

4. **Transportation.** In Britain, whose experience in transporting smallpox cases is far greater than any other Western community, transporting cases and suspects has traditionally been carried out in designated ambulances of standard design. The driver and attendant wear protective clothing with the patient on a standard stretcher. No special precautions are taken to prevent the infection escaping during the patient's transfer to and from the ambulance. Even with smallpox, this somewhat casual approach was usually effective and there are very few instances where an ambulance used in this way was suspected as a source of infection.

It might be considered, therefore, that a designated standard ambulance, subject to thorough disinfection, would be adequate and acceptable for transporting patients suffering from the very much less infectious Lassa or Ebola-Marburg fevers and even pneumonic plague, provided that simple precautions were taken to ensure the filtration of exhausted air. There is little doubt that such a procedure would be safe in the great majority of instances and is i fact practiced in the UK. Other countries, however, notably Australia and Canada, have adopted more stringent precautions utilizing plastic stretcher isolators which achieve the patient's complete isolation from the outside environment during the entire transportation procedure. It seems likely that this practice will eventually be adopted in the UK. The Canadian Armed Forces, in collaboration with Vickers Medical, have developed an isolator for stretcher transportation in road vehicles and a larger model for use in Hercules aircraft.

Although these measures may seem excessive in view of the nature of the diseases which they are designed to transport, their general adoption will probably be ensured by political pressures. These measures will at least ensure safety in the future if other dangerous diseases appear with truly high person-to-person transmissibility.

5. **Contact tracing and surveillance.** Contract tracing and surveillance form an essential part of any public health response and can be modified to suit the threat from any particular disease entity. A critical factor is that under present world conditions, communicable diseases are no longer either parochial or even national in their impact and once international and intercontinental air travel are involved, contact-tracing can become a formidable task. In theory, it should be relatively simple for commercial carriers to keep accurate passenger lists with declared destinations, but in practice, the logistics and costs involved have, in most instances, defeated any such attempt. Passenger lists are retained for no more than four days and are in any case of limited value since they do not give destinations and show only original bookings rather than who actually travelled. In major international airports, with large numbers of stand-by and staging passengers, these omissions seriously reduce the value of passenger lists in contact tracing. The cost of extracting their full potential value by using landing cards would be prohibitive especially in view of the infrequency

with which such information is needed. The entire concept of 'facilitation' in air transport runs counter to the public health requirements. It seems inevitable that contact tracing will remain a retrospective exercise of considerable difficulty.

The tracing and categorization of contacts would be needed with any of the designated diseases but subsequent measures might well differ. Lassa and Ebola fevers and smallpox are alike in that infected contacts do not themselves become infectious until after the onset of clinical illness. They need not, therefore, be segregated in quarantine provided that they are subject to daily personal surveillance throughout the possible incubation period and are isolated immediately if they develop fever or other symptoms or signs of illness. With Lassa and Ebola, only close contacts need be placed under daily surveillance. Close contacts have been defined by the Canadian Contingency Plan[168] as:

(a) members of the patient's household;
(b) people who work closely with the patient;
(c) people who have similar degrees of contact to both (a) and (b);
(j) people who attend the patient during his illness;
(e) people who have direct contact with the patient's blood, urine or secretions;
(f) people who handle the patient's clothing, bedding or other personal belongings;
(g) people who have contact with the corpse.[168]

More remote contacts are at little risk and need only be advised to consult their family doctor if they show signs of illness during the subsequent 21 days.

In smallpox, the net must be cast wider. The variola virus is very stable, resistant to drying and transmissible by the airborne route to remote contacts. A much wider range of contacts must be considered to be at risk. Fortunately, vaccination carried out during the early incubation period provides a high degree of protection and may be combined with surveillance to establish a *cordon sanitaire* around identified cases. The 'Ring-Vaccination' procedure which vaccinates all traceable contacts of the index case as well as all *their* secondary contacts, uses this combination. It has been conspicuously successful in controlling smallpox outbreaks which result from sporadic introductions of the disease, while exposing the risks inherent in the vaccination procedure itself to a minimum number of the population.

In pneumonic plague, experience of appropriate procedures is totally lacking. Contact tracing and surveillance would certainly need to be no less extensive than those for smallpox and should probably also require quarantine of contacts. It is likely that the use of prophylactic anti-bacterials would prove to be a key measure in control.

To be used effectively, these medical measures require smoothly running and efficient community health administration to direct and control the public health response. Contingency planning is required to establish alert and notification channels, consultant services, transporation, hospitalization, contact tracing and surveillance together with media relation and information services.

6. **Public relations.** Public relations including media relations are a major concern in the public health response, partly because of the readiness with which the media can fire a spark of concern into a near-panic, and partly because contact tracing must depend in large measure on media cooperation.

Control and containment in the hospital

The interests of the patient and the requirements of public health come into the most direct conflict in the hospital setting. It is here that the patient will be lodged at the height of his illness when he is at his most infectious and when the problems of containment are most difficult.

The objectives of containment are the localization of the infective agent followed by its total eradication. The slaughter policy of agriculture seeks to achieve these objectives in the most direct manner and even the most rigid isolation procedures when applied in the human setting are already a compromise with safety. In its most extreme form isolation is the total sealing off of a patient from the external environment and the ending of all human contact – a practice seen occasionally during the Black Death in the fourteenth century.[153] From isolation each step which permits progressively greater human contact with the patient represents a further compromise with safety. At the other end of the scale, the lowest grade of 'isolation' procedure is reached when a patient is 'barrier-nursed' in an open multiple-bed ward.

Clearly, the more dangerous the disease the less compromise with safety is acceptable, so little human contact with the patient can be permitted and the conflict between the interests of the patient and the isolation requirement becomes more critical. The period when isolation must be most rigidly applied is precisely the period when the patient is in the greatest danger – when his life may hang upon the promptness and skill with which nursing and life-support procedures can be applied. At this time he will also present the worst problems in patient management and the most dangerous infective hazard to staff caring for him. Nurses must manage the problems of recurrent and uncontrollable diarrhoea, vomiting and pharyngeal and laryngeal obstruction complicated by haemorrhage in a patient who may be in a state of prostration or suffering manic delirium requiring physical restraint – this in full knowledge that an accident may culminate in their own deaths as well as the escape of the infective agent. Diagnosis can be established only by laboratory procedures which involve the examination of blood, stool, pharyngeal secretions and, possibly, serous effusions with attendant risk to staff who collect, handle and examine the specimens. Optimal clinical management demands repeated biochemical and haematological investigations and, almost certainly, invasive therapeutic techniques such as intravenous and, possibly, central venous catheterization, and tracheostomy. Surgical intervention may also be considered necessary.

The conflict of interest is obvious and may be simply stated as: the safer the isolation procedure, the greater the danger to the patient. The better the patient care, the greater the danger to attendant staff and the greater the chance of escape of the infective agent.

Determining an isolation policy demands striking a balance between the risks to the patient and the risks to the community – including the staff caring for the patient – and the selection of an acceptable compromise. This selection must entail a conscious decision as to the practical limit of care which may be given to the patient in view of the attendant hazard to staff and community.

Objectives of isolation

In the hospital the objectives of patient isolation are: localization of the infective agent within a specified area; protection of people outside that area and the ecosystem; and protection of the attendant staff. These two objectives and the techniques and procedures available for their attainment overlap to a great extent but are by no means identical.

Localization of the infective agent

In theory, the localization of the infective agent can be simply achieved by completely enclosing the patient and all potentially infectious materials, including contaminated fomites, excreta, dejecta, effluents and air, together with everyone who has entered the isolation zone and are therefore potentially contaminated within a specified area. The isolation enclosure must be constructed to prevent the escape of any such material.

In practice, this simple ideal cannot be achieved since many of the materials such as soiled clothing and linen, contaminated dressings, excreta, sanitary effluents and air, must be removed from the isolation zone and attendant staff must be permitted movement in and out of the area. Compromises are unavoidable. These too are simple in theory. All that is needed is that non-living materials are sterilized before removal and that staff wear clothing which prevents contamination and which can be discarded when they leave the area. In practice, however, the situation is much more complex. *In situ* sterilization of potentially infective materials is not practical and means must be devised for their safe removal to some other locality where they may be incinerated, autoclaved or otherwise disposed of without permitting contamination. This involves placing solid articles, which are to be removed, within a sealed container whose outside surfaces are uncontaminated or can be decontaminated as it leaves the isolation zone. The entire container and contents are then sterilized or destroyed without opening the container.

This simple solution requires much ingenuity for its implementation and is very susceptible to error. The most frequently employed procedure is that of 'double bagging'. A nurse, within the contaminated zone, places the material to be discarded within a plastic bag which she then 'seals' or, to be more precise, closes by folding over and tying its neck, before taking it to the door of the patient's room and placing it within a second bag held by another nurse who remains outside the room. The second nurse then 'seals' the outer bag, which is outwardly uncontaminated and may be removed from the area. The first bag may additionally be swabbed down with disinfectant before being placed in the outer bag, which may be held open by a mechanical device rather than a second nurse.

No matter what refinements are added, it is clear that such a procedure cannot be made totally safe. The first bag cannot be filled without some external contamination especially around the neck where the folds from closing will protect contaminants from disinfectant however thoroughly this may be applied. Disinfectants do not act instantaneously and nothing short of total immersion in a strong disinfectant solution could ensure disinfection of even the exposed surface. Transferring the first bag through the room door and placing it within the second bag opens the way for airborne contamination to escape and requires the close apposition of contaminated with uncontaminated staff. The provision of ante-rooms and airlocks can reduce but not eliminate this risk. Airlocks are effective only if they are built with adequate air extraction and are used with meticulous procedures.

Most solid materials can be disposed of with reasonable safety using the double bagging procedure; the room air can be extracted through HEPA (High Efficiency Particulate Air) filters which will ensure its safety for external release.

Liquids present additional problems since urine must be regarded as infective and liquids used for cleansing the patient will also contain the infective agent. These fluids must not go through the sewage system without sterilization but no truly satisfactory method for their disposal has yet been devised other than a system of heat treatment to render them sterile before discharge. Such treatment needs a specially designed plant and is not generally available. Three alternative methods are usually employed. The least satisfactory is probably that of bagging the liquids and sending them for autoclaving or incinerating in the liquid state. Apart from the difficulties of handling, the method presents dangers which should be avoided. In some institutions, *in situ* sterilization is used, hypochlorite or formalin is added and the mixture is allowed to stand overnight before being emptied into the sewage system. The third method is to soak up the liquid into some absorbent material which can then be handled as a solid carrier without danger of spillage. This method is the most convenient but is easily applicable only to small volumes of fluid.

With attendant staff, the problems are even greater since there is no way sterilization of even the external surfaces of the body can be achieved. Normal isolation procedures do not call for total enclosure of the staff member in an impermeable covering and the protective clothing normally worn. It is intended only to prevent contamination reaching the underlying clothing which is considered 'clean' when the outer gown is discarded when the person leaves the isolation room. Even in the more stringent procedures, when fully disposable clothing is worn, the body of the staff member is exposed to relatively free circulation of room air and therefore to contamination. Without this ventilation conditions will rapidly become intolerable, and full protection by enclosure within impermeable protective clothing demands some personal ventilation system. Finally, no standard protective clothing completely covers the head, so that the person's face and neck are usually exposed. Surgical masks do little to reduce this exposure or even protect against inhalation of infectious particles. The final discarding of the clothing at the end of a nursing session with the patient also presents a series of problems regarding the possible carry-over of contamination and the danger of generating secondary aerosols from the clothing. These may not only lead to external escape of infection but may present an inhalation hazard to the staff member during disrobing.

Even showering before finally leaving the isolation area cannot be regarded as completely satisfactory. First, it is not a normal practice, even for so-called 'full' isolation, and second, female staff will very rarely wash their hair as a part of their standard showering practice. Unless the clothing worn provides full covering for the head and neck, this leaves a serious loophole in the containment procedure.

Detailed analysis would reveal many more gaps in the supposed isolation techniques usually employed by hospitals, but enough has been said to indicate their inadequacy and to identify the type of problem which is encountered at all points of the interface between the contaminated zone and the 'clean' external environment. Under the conditions described 'isolation' becomes not an absolute but a quantitative phenomenon, where the degree of contamination escaping from the patient's environment is drastically reduced but not entirely eliminated. This fact is tacitly recognized by inclusion of ante-rooms acknowledged as 'grey areas' between the contaminated zone and the 'clean' external environment. With most of the infections common to the Western world, the reduction of contamination achieved by these imperfect techniques is enough to control the spread of infection, because the minimal infective dose of most of the infective agents concerned is relatively large. In very few diseases is the dose required less than 100 viable organisms and even then the dose must penetrate to a susceptible site in the new potential host who must be susceptible to infection. If the numbers of organisms escaping are sufficiently reduced, the statistical chances of engendering a new infection in the external community become small enough for control to be effective.

Typhoid fever is a case in point. Typhoid fever was one of the great epidemic scourges of the past but the minimal infective dose of the causative bacterium, *Salmonella typhi*, is large, in the order of 10,000 viable organisms.[169] Infective bacteria are shed in the stool and in the urine of the infected patient so that airborne contamination is secondary and of low degree. Infection occurs exclusively by the alimentary tract as a result of ingestion of viable bacteria. If stools and urine are carefully handled and sterilized, small numbers of organisms, escaping by the air or by external contamination of fomites, are unlikely to be ingested by a susceptible recipient outside the isolation area in sufficient numbers to cause infection. Typhoid fever is, in fact, one of the easiest diseases to control in a hospital setting since person-to-person spread can be prevented by simple hygienic behaviour.

By contrast, smallpox requires the most stringent precautions for adequate control. Infection occurs by the respiratory route and, by analogy with the closely allied vaccinia and rabbit-pox viruses, a single viable particle of the causative variola virus is sufficient to initiate infection.[7] The virus is shed from the skin in enormous quantities from ruptured vesicles and pustules during the eruptive phase of the disease, the bloodstained exudates saturate the patient's clothing and bed-linen from which massive secondary aerosols can be derived through the slightest disturbance. In certain patients a variolous pneumonia may lead to the generation of a primary aerosol derived directly from the respiratory secretions. These patients are very infectious.

The virus itself is extremely stable. It is resistant to inactivation by drying and remains infectious for a long time in air or room dust from which secondary aerosols may be derived. In 1948 in the UK, two painters contracted smallpox while redecorating a smallpox hospital. The hospital had been closed for two years since the last case of smallpox had been nursed there. Subsequently, variola virus was recovered from room dust sweepings from beneath the floor through which debris from the patients' skin had penetrated. Clearly, that under such conditions absolute containment must be the goal and the penalties for failure may be severe as seen in the 1961–62 outbreak of smallpox in Britain,[6, 7] the Meschede Hospital incident in West Germany,[5] the laboratory breaks at the London School of Hygiene in 1973 and Birmingham University in 1978.

High security isolation

With diseases as dangerous as smallpox, the normal facilities and procedures are grossly inadequate and the requirements need to be considered *de novo* in relation to both containment and staff protection under the following headings:

1. **Functions**. An isolation facility should provide the structural basis for certain definable functions. It must provide for

   (a) safe access to and from the exterior;
   (b) 'clean' administrative functions;
   (c) patient isolation and treatment;
   (d) safe transition between (b) and (c);
   (e) removal of contaminated materials, and of corpses in the event of death;
   (f) safe disposal of liquid effluent;

(g) sterilization of discharged air;

(h) prevention of unintentional or accidental leakage of air or fluids;

(i) easy disinfection of all contaminated areas;

(j) back-up for all mechanisms essential for safe operation.

To satisfy these requirements, five basic zones are required although the degree of elaboration within each may be varied within wide limits. The requirements outlined below may be regarded as the minimum for complete safety.

2. **Structure.** For maximum safety, any high security isolation facility should preferably be located in open country well away from major populated areas. It should be housed in a building exclusively for this purpose and physically separated from any other building, particularly if the facility is built in association with an existing hospital or university medical school. Access to it should be separate from access to any other building. Its air supply and ventilation system should be separate from that of any other building and all discharged air should first be filtered through HEPA filters to an extraction efficiency of 99.97 per cent at 0.3 μm particle size as assessed by the DOP test method. Liquid effluent derived from contaminated or potentially contaminated areas should be heat-sterilized before discharge. The building should contain an autoclave and an incinerator for the sterilization and disposal of contaminated materials. Walls, floors and ceilings should be made of impermeable, durable and corrosion-resistant materials. There should be no hanging ceilings.

The interior of the building should be divided into five physically defined zones.

- *An outer clean zone* with direct access to the exterior. This zone should have staff changing rooms, inward access through a one-way door to the second zone and outward access from that zone through a shower.
- *An inner clean zone* housing the administrative function, nursing station, rest and relaxation rooms.
- *A safety zone* separating the inner clean zone from the isolation zone. This zone should contain two ante-rooms arranged in series and separated by an airlock and shower. These would

be duplicated for male and female staff. The outer ante-rooms should be 'clean' while the inner, in direct contact with the isolation zone, would be potentially contaminated.

- *An isolation zone* containing the patient treatment area. Besides the requisite number of patient rooms, this zone should provide a nursing service area giving access to 'clean' and 'dirty' utility rooms. The dirty utility room should contain the inner end of a pass-through autoclave where all contaminated materials for disposal should be sterilized before being incinerated or discarded.
- *A plant zone* containing the mechanical plant required for the facility. Access should be from outside the building by a distinct entrance so that maintenance staff can operate and service the machinery without entering the main part of the building. The outer end of the pass-through autoclave should open into a part of this area adjacent to the incinerator.

Provision must be made for admitting patients directly into the isolation zone without going through the clean zones, and for the removal of corpses.

In all zones, and particularly at all zone interfaces, appropriate directional airflow must be established so that under all conditions air travels only from the less to the more contaminated region.

Designing such a building is not easy and its use would inevitably be cumbersome and expensive. The structure itself does not protect the personnel caring for the patient. This protection must be achieved by means of appropriate equipment and procedures.

3. **Protecting staff – equipment and procedures.** Protective equipment is intended to isolate the health-care staff from the patient and his contaminated environment. This result may be achieved either by isolating the staff from the patient or the patient from the staff. The former method relies upon using protective clothing which, ideally, totally encloses the staff member in a clean, protected bubble which permits safe functioning in the contaminated environment.

Isolating the patient from the staff is a more recent technique, developed from the life-island concept, where the patient is totally enclosed within a sealed environment – basically a complex plastic bag – which confines the contaminated zone into a small area. The staff member does not penetrate this area. The only access is by invaginations in the plastic envelope of the isolator.

Protective clothing to be effective under conditions where the danger of infection is great must ensure complete coverage of the body, including skin and conjunctiva, and must ensure that the air breathed is sterile. The classical cotton gown with surgical mask and gloves is inadequate for this purpose.

Good protection may be achieved wearing a 'jump-suit' type of garment made from impermeable material with tight cuffs overlapped by rubber gloves, snug closure at the neck over a cape extension of a complete hood, and a whole-face respirator fitted with a bacterial filter. This complete enclosure within impermeable materials, gives rise to overheating problems and the clothing cannot be worn for long periods.

More recently, plastic suits have been designed, usually as two-piece garments. The tunic ties at the waist and the person's head is completely enclosed within a head-piece which is a continuation of the tunic. Air is fed into the head-piece either by an 'umbilical' tube from outside the contaminated area or by a portable battery-operated fan-filter unit integral with the suit (see Figures 5a and 5b).

The chief advantage of this system lies in its flexibility. In its simplest form, the cotton gown with surgical mask and gloves interferes very little with patient care; it is easily upgraded by using a hood, face-shield and disposable tunic and trousers together with surgical-type disposable gown with waterproof front surface. The system is acceptable to nursing staff and it is inexpensive. Nursing teams could rapidly be expanded to manage even large outbreaks without seriously straining resources.

The main disadvantage is that protection is less than complete, particularly against respiratory infection and body contamination unless a gas-mask type full-face respirator and impermeable clothing are worn.

The more sophisticated mechanically ventilated plastic suits give full protection. They permit most medical and nursing procedures with little interference, are cool and well-protected and relatively inexpensive. The umbilical type involves trailing

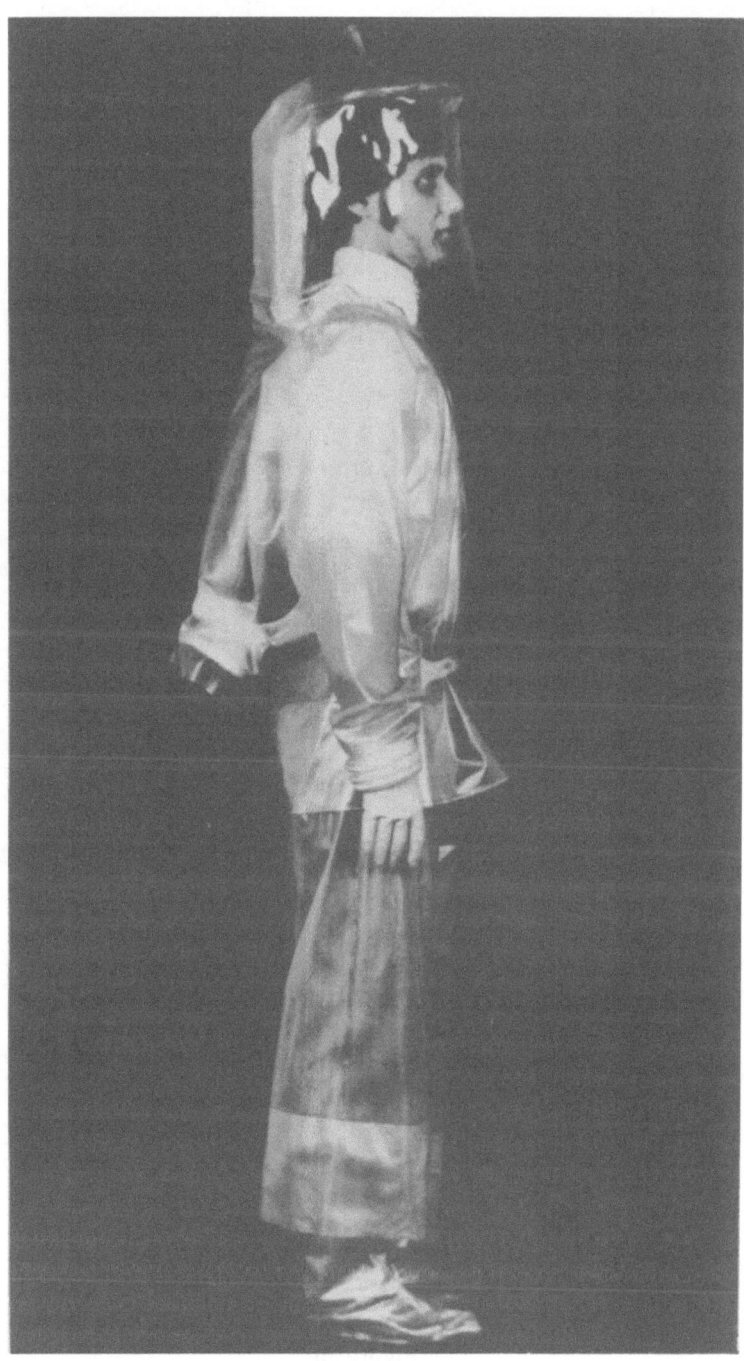

Figure 5a

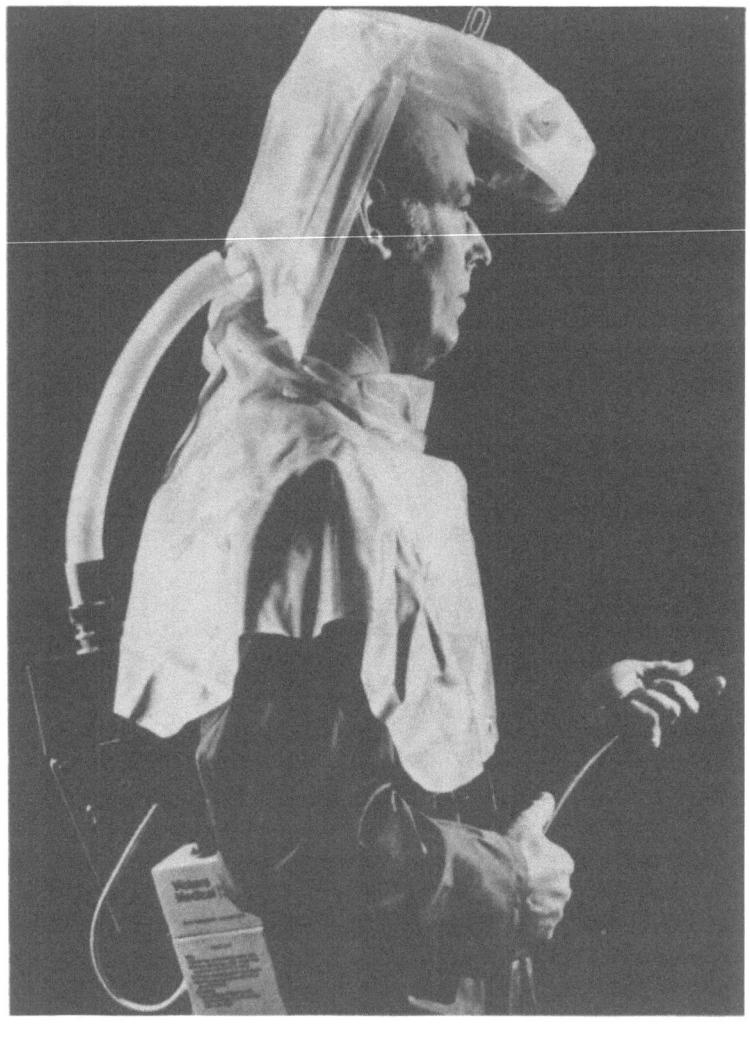

Figure 5b

a length of tubing, which can be a nuisance especially if there is more than one staff member present. The types using portable fan-filter units vary in weight and noise-level but some are well within acceptable limits.

Ventilated hoods and suits have been used for protection against inhalation of radioactive dust and have proved satisfactory but need more development if they are to be used against exotic diseases. The units are relatively inexpensive and require little training to use so that in an emergency, provision could quickly be made for the management of numerous patients in an improvised isolation area.

There are problems though. A person wearing a ventilated hood cannot use auscultation and devising an adequate procedure for its external decontamination and discarding at the end of a duty period is also a problem. In the UK there is an additional problem since ethylene oxide sterilization is not acceptable. This problem would not arise in Canada or the US. Failure of the ventilation units has been known to occur.

The plastic patient isolator reverses the isolation procedure and encloses the patient instead of the staff member. To date only a single type has been produced. The patient is totally enclosed within a strong plastic envelope which is supported by a metal frame. Filtered air is supplied from the room where the patient bed isolator (PBI) is located and exhaust air is evacuated through a HEPA filter to the outside. The ventilation system is balanced to ensure that the interior of the isolator is maintained at a negative pressure relative to the room air (see Figure 6).

The outstanding advantage of the plastic bed isolator is that it precisely demarcates and encloses the contaminated area, and gives complete protection against all mechanisms of transmission. Consequently, not only do the attendant staff know exactly where the contaminated area ends but, if they are outside it, they do not need to take any special protective measures such as wearing protective clothing. As long as the isolator remains intact and functional, they are completely protected. In the circumstances surrounding these lethal diseases, this gives a tremendous psychological advantage.

A second advantage lies in the great simplification achieved in the structural requirements of the isolation facility. Theoretically, the only requirement is a room large enough to

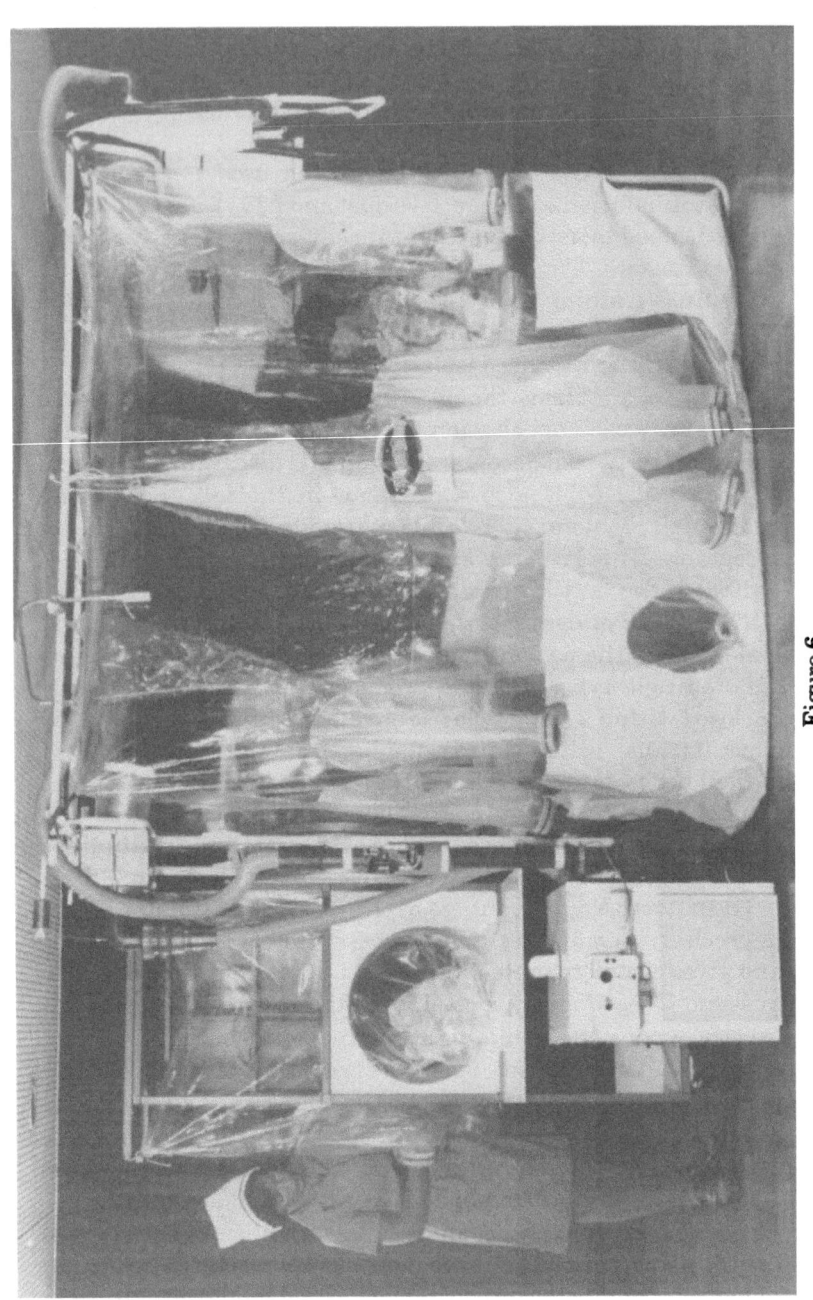

Figure 6

house the erected isolator and its ancillary equipment. In practice, elementary prudence demands additional measures, but these are relatively simple since the total enclosure of the patient and his contaminated environment eliminates the need for both the isolation zone and for the complex safety zone described above. The requirement is reduced to an outer clean zone, a plant zone, and an inner clean zone, incorporating the nursing service area and rooms containing the bed-isolators.

Although these structural requirements should be met in any permanent, purpose-designed isolation facility, the fact that the isolator can be safely used without them means that in an emergency, one or more could be flown, together with trained staff, to any threatened locality and set up in any room large enough to hold them. This emergency potential could be extremely valuable.

The main disadvantages of the bed-isolator lie in the cumbersome nature of the procedures required for patient management and maintenance of the integrity of the system when introducing or removing materials, and in the limitation which it imposes on practical measures of patient care. Access to the patient is by invaginations in the plastic envelope which end in heavy-gauge gloves and requires wearing a ventilated waistcoat and head-harness to support the weight of the plastic pocket. Rapid access to the patient is difficult and problems could arise from patients who are delirious or who would not tolerate the enclosure. Similarly, persistent vomiting and diarrhoea would not be easy to manage. It is also possible that in an emergency such as acute laryngeal obstructions which require emergency tracheostomy, the need for fast access to the patient might necessitate slashing open the isolator.

Finally, the procedures required for safe use of the isolator are complex and are not a simple extension of familiar nursing procedures. Special training is required for both medical and nursing staff. Consequently, the system is relatively inflexible and is incapable of rapid expansion to cope with many patients, limited by the number of isolators and trained teams available.

4. **Procedures.** Whether the system of staff or patient enclosure is used, the effectiveness of any equipment is absolutely dependent upon the meticulous use of appropriate procedures. In this respect, North America generally is at a disadvantage to

the UK since its health-care systems do not include isolation hospitals whose basic function is the safe management of infectious diseases. In such hospitals, isolation technique is a way of life rather than a special procedure. Without this advantage of habituation, it is imperative for safety that staff be trained with examplary thoroughness.

12

Appropriate Level of Response

The problem of response is divisible into three issues: the public health response in the community at large; the requirement for special isolation facilities and high security laboratories; and the measures to be taken in general hospitals.

Response in the community

The public health response as it affects the community at large is aimed at limiting the spread of infection by means of rapid detection and segregation of cases, and tracing and surveillance of contacts.

Efficient working depends largely on good contingency planning backed by good information gathering and dissemination at the national level and an effective public health personnel structure. For fast and effective response, the sequences of alert, notification and action and the channels to be followed must be known and observed – this is largely a matter of forethought and good administration. The medical problems are detection, diagnosis and immediate patient management when suspicion is aroused, the immediate need being segregation. The main difficulty is to strike a balance between caution and practicality and this demands an understanding of the transmissibility and mechanisms of transmission of the disease suspected – an understanding which is far from universal among physicians.

Once segregation has been achieved, the problem in the community then shifts to contact-tracing and management.

Contact tracing is a matter of patient detective work and management, fortunately, is simplified by the facts that close contact is required for transmission and infected persons do not become infectious until after clinical onset. Close contacts may be classified according to the criteria adopted from the UK Memorandum on Lassa Fever, and incorporated into the Canadian Contingency Plan.[168] Close contacts require daily surveillance with immediate segregation if they become ill. More remote contacts do not require active surveillance but should be instructed to consult their physician if they become ill.

2. Special isolation facilities

In terms of hospital isolation facilities and procedures, the five diseases which need to be considered require, from the scientific point of view, widely different levels of response.

Smallpox and pneumonic plague must be treated as highly communicable diseases with a major potential for community spread by respiratory person-to-person transmission. Variola virus also presents a danger of spread by contaminated fomites. Containing both diseases requires the most stringent precautions. On the other hand, hospital staff can be effectively protected against smallpox by vaccination and against plague by chemoprophylaxis. The dominant problem is containment.

By contrast, Lassa fever has minimal potential for person-to-person spread. The same is true of Ebola-Marburg fever despite the apparent contradiction of the Sudan and Zaire episodes. The evidence strongly suggests that neither of these diseases could cause community epidemics in developed communities. On the other hand, both diseases are transmissible by close physical contact, especially to persons caring for patients at the height of their illness, and so pose a dangerous threat of nosocomial infection to staff. In the community, they are among the least infectious of virus diseases and require no more than standard isolation procedures for their control. Within the hospital, their lethality demands that the most stringent precautions are taken for the protection of attendant staff.

Yellow fever is also not transmitted directly from person-to-person so does not pose a threat of community spread outside the geographical distribution of its vector, nor does it appear to be a danger to attendant staff although several investigators have died as a result of laboratory-acquired infection. Isolation for this disease is required only in regions where the *Aedes aegypti* or other potential vector is present and must then be aimed at protection from mosquito-bite for the short period during which viraemia is present.

While the simple and probably the most logical answer to the problem of selecting an appropriate level of response would be to cater for the most demanding diseases – smallpox and plague – on the ground that this would automatically ensure an adequate response to the less demanding diseases, there are practical objections to this course of action.

First is the expense. Isolation facilities incorporating the full requirements are expensive to build and operate, and, as discussed earlier, this requirement is likely to be self-defeating. The inhibitory action of the prospective cost is reinforced by other considerations. The operation of such an elaborate facility is inevitably cumbersome and time-consuming for health-care staff and also requires continuous mechanical and structural maintenance. Although it would be difficult to use the facility for less dramatic purposes it would be not only uneconomic but also impractical to permit it to stand idle between crises. It would be unrealistic to expect either the health-care and operating procedures or the elaborate mechanical plant to function perfectly on the basis of sporadic utilization. On-going training and continued usage would be an unavoidable requirement for effectiveness when stringent isolation is required.

To this must be added a further consideration. Of the two diseases which demand such stringent measures for their containment against community epidemic spread, smallpox has now been officially eradicated and pneumonic plague appears to be more of a theoretical than actual threat in most areas of the world – even in regions where the disease is endemic. In North America, the threat has never materialized since it was introduced into California at the beginning of this century.

It would seem that the public health response should be adjusted to the level required for controlling and containing Lassa and Ebola-Marburg fevers.

The possibility of epidemic re-emergence of Ebola-Marburg

fever in Africa cannot be gauged. Without an epidemic, the probability of its introduction into Canada by a human case is less than that of Lassa fever which has an extensive endemic incidence. The possibility of its introduction in a batch of monkeys imported for experimental purposes will, however, remain.

Lassa fever, on the other hand, is a continuing threat. The introduction of cases into North America is certain to continue and requires a positive response.

Since these diseases are characterized by low person-to-person transmissibility and little potential for community spread, the problem of containment takes second place to protecting health-care staff including laboratory personnel. To achieve this, no elaborate facilities are actually needed. Theoretically, standard isolation facilities even within the confines of a functioning hospital would ensure containment and nursing and medical staff could be adequately protected by the standard isolation procedures. Protection of laboratory staff would also be based largely on appropriate policies and procedures regarding specimen taking, but would also require safety equipment and techniques beyond those normally used in hospital diagnostic laboratories.

Although adopting this simple level of response can be defended on the basis of the known facts, more stringent precautions are required because of the fear engendered by the two diseases and because the possibility of respiratory transmission cannot be ruled out. This type of spread may already have occurred with Lassa fever in the Jos hospital outbreak.

When the possibilities of mutation towards higher transmissibility in the two known diseases and the future emergence of yet other diseases with unknown capabilities are also considered, it is clear that special measures exceeding standard isolation procedures are a political and social necessity. A logical response is, however, certainly impossible to achieve in terms of balancing cost, both in money and effort, against risk. Apart from laboratory infections, not a single case of either disease has occurred outside the endemo-epidemic areas of Africa and the risk does not begin to compare with that of influenza which is accepted with no more than transient annual interest. Fear of the unknown escalates the response level needed to an unrealistic but unavoidable degree.

There is no purpose in speculating what future measures should be taken if either disease acquires the transmissibility of influenza since there would then be no possibility of control or containment. With a more modest degree of respiratory transmissibility, containment would be a more realistic goal due to the rarity of importation. Even in the UK, which has been the country most heavily exposed, all the introductions have been single events and not more than one individual at a time has had to be isolated as a serious suspect. Under these conditions, the plastic bed isolator and the ventilated protective suit provide acceptable, practical and relatively inexpensive alternatives. Their respective merits and demerits in relation to patient management may be restated as they affect public health response.

The plastic bed-isolator. Provided that not more than a few cases require isolation at any one time, the plastic bed-isolator provides the most comprehensive basis for an adequate response because of the following:

(1) It affords complete containment so it gives effective protection against all types of transmission except direct accidental inoculation.
(2) It may be housed in a permanent isolation facility of simple design which would be relatively inexpensive to build and operate. If desired, several such facilities could be built to disperse isolation capacity. This has already been done in the UK.
(3) In an emergency it can be flown with a trained team to any part of the country and set up in any room large enough to hold it.
(4) It is relatively inexpensive.

Although theoretically the isolator assures complete containment if correctly used, the procedures for introducing and removing objects, for example instruments or specimens for laboratory examination, are elaborate and specialized and are not a straightforward extension of normal nursing technique. It has, therefore, been tacitly accepted that the isolator should be housed in a purpose-designed isolation facility which can be of simpler design than previously described. A separate building or wing with access through changing rooms and showers would still be desirable; within the building the patient treatment area would not need to be segregated from the clean zone although individual isolators might be housed in separate glass-walled cubicles, each exhaust-ventilated, but opening into a common utility room.

Contaminated materials are removed from the isolator by passing them into a plastic invagination which is then sealed off by ligaturing its neck and cutting through between ligatures with an electric soldering iron which melts the plastic and simultaneously heat-sterilizes the cut surface. The outer surface of the bag is uncontaminated and can be removed from the isolation area with safety so that autoclaving before removal to an incinerator is not required and the incinerator need not be an integral part of the isolation facility. The cost of a building of this type is less than one-fifth of a full-scale, purpose-designed facility incorporating the five zones required.

Ventilated protective suits. The alternative to isolating the patient in an elaborate plastic bag is to isolate each member of the health-care staff in a ventilated plastic bubble (see Figures 5a and 5b) which may be a complete suit if it is necessary to protect the entire body, or may be restricted to a hood covering the head and neck to the shoulders if only respiratory protection is needed. This hood is all that is needed with the diseases now under consideration since the body can be effectively protected by disposable gown and gloves. Ventilation is by air pumped into the head-covering either through a flexible tube originating outside the contaminated area or by a portable battery-driven, fan-filter unit carried on the person's body. While these units vary in weight, comfort and noise-level, all are practical and can be worn continuously for two hours or more without distress. They permit the free performance of all patient-management procedures with the single exception of auscultation.

The advantages of this type of personal protection are that normal nursing and patient-management procedures can be carried out, so special training is not required; there is little or no interference with patient care, and emergency intervention is possible; the system is psychologically more acceptable to the patient; the equipment is not expensive and maintaining a large reserve capacity is not a major problem, so the capacity of a facility could be rapidly expanded and mobility is greater than the bed-isolator.

The main disadvantages are that since contamination is not rigidly contained within a small defined area a more elaborate structural facility is needed than for the bed-isolator. In consequence, this complete containment could not be established except in locations where purpose-designed facilities were available. This might limit its acceptability as a mobile technique in small towns or remote areas. Safe removal, disposal and disinfection of the suit and fan-filter unit raises procedural problems.

Both systems have their advantages and disadvantages and both systems are in use in different institutions. In the UK the bed-isolator is used in Bristol at the Ham Green Hospital, in Manchester at the Monsall Hospital, in London at Coppetts Wood Hospital and in Glasgow at the Ruchill Hospital. It has also been adopted in Canada at the National Defence Medical Centre in Ottawa and in Australia at the Fairfield Hospital, Melbourne.

The ventilated suit technique has been developed at the General Hospital, Newcastle-upon-Tyne. At the Fazakerley Hospital, Liverpool, primary reliance is placed upon the bed-isolator but ventilated hoods are held in reserve and would permit rapid expansion into a series of cubicles which have been included within the high-security isolation wing. This combination, taking advantage of the virtues of both systems, would seem to be the best approach now available.

3. The general hospital

The general community hospital is likely to become involved in the exotic disease problem at two different levels. The first and most obvious is that patients with pyrexias of unknown origin are likely to be admitted before a suspicion of Lassa or Ebola arises so that the hospital must eventually respond to a *fait accompli*. The second is that the number of suspect cases who do not have either of these diseases will greatly outnumber the cases where the suspicion is ultimately confirmed. The management of suspects may therefore be a not infrequent requirement in certain hospitals.

Isolation requirements. It is likely that there is no general community hospital at the present time which could safely isolate a case of smallpox. Paradoxically, the more modern the hospital the less it is capable of establishing effective isolation. This stems from the modern architectural concepts of 'open plan' design, service floors extending over whole wings, elevator shafts and suspended ceilings often with absorbent acoustic tiles. The need to close an entire 500-bed modern general hospital in Toronto to isolate one suspected case of Lassa fever in 1976, and the inability to fumigate the Microbiology Laboratory at the Children's Hospital of Eastern Ontario because an entire hospital floor, including the operating rooms, would be gassed in the process, support this statement.

Fortunately, Lassa and Ebola fevers do not require more than the standard isolation procedures now practiced in most hospitals for their containment, and these could be reinforced at relatively short notice by the plastic bed-isolator. The danger of community infections occurring, even from unrecognized cases, is small but there would be a real danger of transference of infection to other patients in the hospital and the danger to attendant staff and laboratory personnel would be formidable.

To counter these dangers, two steps are needed. First, all general hospitals should give immediate positive thought to the physical, procedural and laboratory problems of isolation within their own settings.

The following guidelines represent the best results to be achieved in a general hospital setting and it is appreciated that few hospitals could achieve the physical requirements described which alone would permit the suggested procedures to be followed.

Certain hospitals are in a particularly vulnerable position. They will often receive patients of many different nationalities who have recently arrived from many areas of the world. For them, the necessary expenditure for planning, modification and/or *de novo* building should be seriously considered.

For less exposed hospitals, these guidelines may serve as a basis from which a compromise course of action may be selected within the prevailing fiscal restraints. When compromises are selected, it must be appreciated that safety procedures are necessarily governed and limited by the physical facilities in which they must operate and by the equipment available. This dependence is given further point by industrial safety legislation in an increasing number of countries which makes it a legal obligation for an employer to establish adequate physical facilities to ensure the safety of staff and to train them in the correct use of those facilities.

Physical problems. The purpose should be to develop or modify physical facilities to the point where they still remain a practical asset in the hospital's normal functioning, but can be instantly converted into a high-security isolation unit which could safely contain both the disease and its respiratory spread. In most instances, this would mean modifying an existing wing or section of a ward large enough to form a useful adjunct to the normal working of the hospital but small enough to be closed up for high-security isolation without seriously reducing the number of beds available for normal use.

Structurally, the isolation unit should provide the following:

(1) the patient room(s);
(2) one, or preferably two, ante-rooms to the patient room(s);
(3) the nursing station;
(4) a staff relaxation room with wash-room and toilet;
(5) a separate ventilation system;
(6) access for staff;
(7) access for patients;
(8) an outlet for disposal of discarded materials, garbage and corpses.

1. *The patient room(s)* should:
(a) have integral floor, walls and ceiling of non-porous materials resistant to disinfectants;
(b) have sealed windows;
(c) have a toilet and wash-room for use only when the room is being used for other than high-security isolation or when the patient is no longer infectious;
(d) be approached through at least one ante-room.

2. *The ante-rooms.* There should be a separate ante-room to each patient room and access should be only through this ante-room. A second, *outer* ante-room should also be provided.

The outer ante-room could serve more than one patient room and would be a general utility area.

The inner ante-room should contain: a series of discard bins with foot-operated lids and plastic sac liners; the liners should be colour coded for disposal method – incineration, autoclaving, re-use etc; the number of bins will be determined by the procedures adopted; facilities for gluteraldehyde disinfection of small instruments and reusable equipment, and for sodium hypochlorite disinfection of containers of specimens for laboratory examination; hand-washing and disinfection facilities; access to the outer ante-room through a shower.

The outer ante-room may serve as a utility area for one or more patient isolation rooms. It should contain: storage space for protective clothing and clean coveralls; hanging space for clothing removed before entry to isolation rooms; space for temporary holding of double-bagged packages removed from isolation rooms and access to disposal area.

3. *The nursing station* should be in a clean area separated by a door from the outer ante-room; have 'intercom' communication with the patient rooms; be placed so that patients in the individual rooms are visible through glass windows and have a rest and relaxation room with wash-room facilities.

4. *The isolation unit* as a whole should be accessible to staff without the need to traverse other patient areas; capable of being effectively closed off from the other patient areas of the hospital; provided with changing rooms where staff may change on arrival and departure from the unit; separated from the changing room by a shower.

5. *Ventilation.* The entire isolation unit should be positively ventilated without recirculation of air; the ventilation system should be separate and not shared with other hospital areas; exhaust air should be filtered to no less than 99 per cent efficiency at $0.3\,\mu m$ as determined by the DOP test, before discharge to the exterior; all windows should be sealed closed and no 'natural' ventilation permitted.

Air input and extraction should be arranged so that the flow of air is always inwards from the nursing station to the patient isolation rooms and never outwards from the patient isolation rooms. This can be simply ensured if air input is restricted to the nursing station (and possibly the outer ante-room) and air extraction is restricted to the patient isolation rooms, an uninterrupted flow of air being maintained through louvred grilles in the intervening doors. To maintain the desired directional air flow, airlocks and balanced pressure differentials should not be relied on.

Procedures

Written procedures should be developed to ensure the following requirements are fulfilled when the unit functions in its high-security mode:

(1) Staff working in the isolation unit must, on arrival, change all clothes, including underwear, for designated working clothes before entering the unit.

(2) Working clothes should be simple and should consist of underwear (disposable if possible), disposable coveralls, and a bonnet to enclose the hair. These should be donned in the outer changing room.

Once clothed, staff may enter the isolation unit but all clothing worn there must be discarded within the unit and incinerated (or autoclaved before laundering in the case of non-disposable items), the staff member returns to the changing room through a shower. At no time should the clothing worn in the isolation unit be worn elsewhere.

(3) Protective clothing. All persons entering a patient isolation room must don full protective clothing in the outer ante-room.

Protective clothing must consist exclusively of good quality, disposable, single-use items and may be based on either a knee-length gown and trouser combination or on a one-piece coverall. Garments should be loose-fitting for coolness and must have effective overlap closures at neck, wrist and ankle. Velcro closures serve this purpose. Garments should have waterproof fronts or plastic aprons should be worn.

The clothing must also include the following:

Hood: either integral with the gown (or coverall) or with a shoulder cape to fit under it, and a snug, overlap closure around the face.

Overshoes: in the form of disposable bootees.

Gloves: of good quality rubber or plastic.

Mask: a full-face mask with a microbial filter may be required or a portable ventilated hood may be used if there is danger of respiratory transmission. Where this degree of protection is not necessary or cannot be provided, a good quality surgical mask should be worn.

Visor: for direct patient contact a clear plastic face-shield on an adjustable head-band support should be worn to prevent droplet contamination of the conjunctiva unless a full-face mask or ventilated hood is used.

These items of protective clothing should be stored in the outer ante-room. They should be donned by attendant staff either over or replacing the coveralls worn to enter the unit.

(4) Discarding protective clothing. Staff should discard all garments in the inner ante-room when they leave the patient isolation room.

Gown, trousers, visor and hood should be discarded in this order, followed by bootees and gloves and under-clothes. The larger items should be turned inside out during disrobing and gently folded to minimize the forma-tion of secondary aerosols. The mask should be worn as a protection against this hazard until all other garments have been removed and discarded.

Disposable garments should be placed into a bin lined with a strong plastic bag colour-coded for incineration. Non-disposable garments should be placed in a similar bin lined with an autoclavable plastic bag.

Plastic visors and other items which would not with-stand heat should be separately bagged for ethylene oxide sterilization or should be immersed in 2 per cent gluteral-dehyde for at least 30 minutes before being rinsed and dried for reuse.

Hands must be thoroughly washed before leaving the inner ante-room through a shower. After showering, clean clothing is donned in the outer ante-room.

(5) Instruments. Non-disposable equipment and instruments capable of withstanding autoclaving should also be treated with gluteraldehyde before being bagged for removal. Non-disposable equipment which cannot be

reliably disinfected should not be used in the isolation rooms.

Much of this work can be carried out by the nurse coming on duty when a staff change is due.

(6) Garbage. All discarded materials and soiled disposable patient gowns and bed clothes should be bagged in the patient's room. The sealed bags should be swabbed down with gluteraldehyde before they are removed to the inner ante-room where they are placed within another plastic bag colour-coded for incineration.

(7) Excreta. When patients are continent, plastic-lined bed-pans or closets should be used and solid faeces bagged for incineration. Liquid faeces and urine should be first absorbed in a suitable absorbent – such as absorbent wool, saw-dust or cat litter – to prevent accidental spillage before being similarly bagged.

Removing material for disposal. All material bagged in the inner ante-room for disposal must be double-bagged for removal from the unit for final disposal. This procedure can best be carried out without contaminating the outer bag at the time of a shift change when the uncontaminated relief nurse and the out-going nurse can work together. Each double-bagged, colour-coded package should be placed in the outer ante-room as soon as it has been closed. After showering and dressing in clean coveralls, the out-going nurse should remove them to the garbage-disposal outlet of the unit. If desired, triple-bagging may be carried out before final removal. This outlet should open off the outer ante-room if possible, otherwise, it must open off the nursing station area.

Leaving the isolation unit. Staff leaving the unit must do so through the unit changing rooms. All clothing worn in the unit must be discarded in an ante-room before the staff member enters a shower to gain access to the changing room where his clothes were originally left.

Conclusion

In this account of physical and procedural requirements, the complexities of ensuring both containment and safety become obvious. The system suggested may seem over-complex but simplification involves compromises which become unacceptable when examined individually.

For example, it is unlikely from the transmission pattern of Lassa fever that clothes worn in the patient isolation room would really cause a spread of infection if a nurse coming off duty walks through the hospital without changing, or even goes home. Should the requirement for an elaborate disrobing procedure therefore be dropped? The logical answer on the scientific evidence is probably yes. But would such a course of action be socially or politically acceptable when considering the potential lethality of the disease? With the exception of pneumonic plague the diseases considered are not usually transmitted by aerial spread. Dilution alone would reduce the probability of infection from unfiltered ventilation discharge to vanishingly small proportions, and in an efficiently ventilated hospital, there is little obvious reason to go to the trouble and expense of separating the ventilation system of the isolation unit from that of the remainder of the hospital.

Is it in fact really necessary to do more than open the window? Again in the context of Lassa or Ebola fevers – probably not. Yet the lessons of the Meschede incident when individuals on three hospital floors were infected with smallpox by a single patient confined to his bed in one ward, and of the transmission of tuberculosis through hospital ventilation systems, make one hesitate to condemn the ventilation requirements outlined as superfluous and expensive luxuries. If transmission actually occurs by whatever means to a staff member or to another patient, and if the infected individual dies, a hospital would find itself in an indefensible position if measures had not been adopted to guard against the known mechanisms by which infectious diseases may be transmitted.

Failure to adopt such measures can only be justified on the ground that the financial burden and the interference with good patient management are too great and consequently a degree of risk of transmission to attendant staff and other patients must be accepted in terms of practicality. It must also be agreed that acceptance of the risk of transmission necessarily also implies acceptance of the risk of death of the infected individuals. Logically there would be no problem in defending such a contention since parallel compromises between known risk and absolute safety are an accepted part of our daily lives, but in practice, the justification would be very difficult.

Handling suspects

The most difficult isolation problem facing community hospitals, however, is not likely to be the isolation of cases but rather defining behaviour regarding suspects. The problem is clearly illustrated in the analyses by Emond and Woodruff and their colleagues.[165, 180] In the former study, examination of sera from 86 travellers returning to Britain from tropical Africa revealed evidence of past infection with 10 different identifiable viruses, but no Lassa antibodies were detected. In the latter, the case histories of 79 patients with PUO referred to Coppett's Wood Hospital were reviewed. Of these, 73 were travellers who had returned from tropical Africa, 19 became ill before their departure for the UK and the remaining 54 developed fever within three weeks of their return. Forty-six of the total number were referred specifically because of suspected viral haemorrhagic fever (VHF).

The essential point is that of the returning travellers, only one proved to have VHF, and this case was admitted to a general ward of a major London teaching hospital where the diagnosis was eventually made before referral to Coppett's Wood. The only other positive case was a laboratory infection with Ebola virus acquired in Britain as the result of a known laboratory accident resulting in direct inoculation of infective material.[111] Most of the remaining cases were suffering from malaria. Of the 46 patients referred for suspected VHF, 15 were admitted to standard isolation, 20 to a 'high-security' room and 11 directly into a bed isolator, illustrating the difficulty in diagnosis even by highly experienced clinicians.

This experience emphasizes the rarity with which VHF is likely to be encountered in most Western countries and the relative frequency of malaria as a cause of PUO. Since prompt treatment of malaria may be life-saving, it is essential that the fear of Lassa or Ebola fevers should not be permitted to delay malarial diagnosis and treatment. This viewpoint has been repeatedly stressed by physicians in charge of the British isolation facilities.

In fact, the problem goes further. Today there are six designated facilities for treating VHF cases in Britain:

1. Coppett's Wood Hospital, London – serving London and the Southeast
2. Ham Green Hospital, Pill, near Bristol – serving the Southwest
3. Monsall Hospital, Manchester and
4. Fazakerley Hospital, Liverpool – serving the Midlands
5. The General Hospital, Newcastle-upon-Tyne – serving the North
6. Ruchill Hospital, Glasgow – serving Scotland

Coppett's Wood Hospital has by far the largest population in its catchment area with traffic from two major airports funnelling into London. Other hospitals in the area are reluctant to inundate the facility with cases so they do not refer cases unless their suspicions are strong. This means that a considerable number of PUO cases recently returned from Africa are retained within these community hospitals for preliminary investigation. The treating physician thinks these patients are unlikely to be infected with VHF – but they may be. How are such patients managed until a diagnosis is made, or alternatively, until the suspicion of VHF crystallizes to the point where referral is justified? According to Professor Lambert of St George's Hospital in the London area[38] this problem is a major concern.

The second requirement, therefore, is for hospitals which are likely to encounter such patients, for instance, in large cities or involved in treating tropical diseases, to formulate a definite policy for their management.

Transporting patients. It is clear from the natural history of Lassa and Ebola fevers that infected patients could be transported by normal ambulance during the first week after onset without risk. After that, the risk to attendant staff would increase as the major clinical manifestations set in. Despite the probable safety of transportation during the early stages after onset, it would be socially and politically unacceptable that the movement of suspect patients should be undertaken without special precautions.

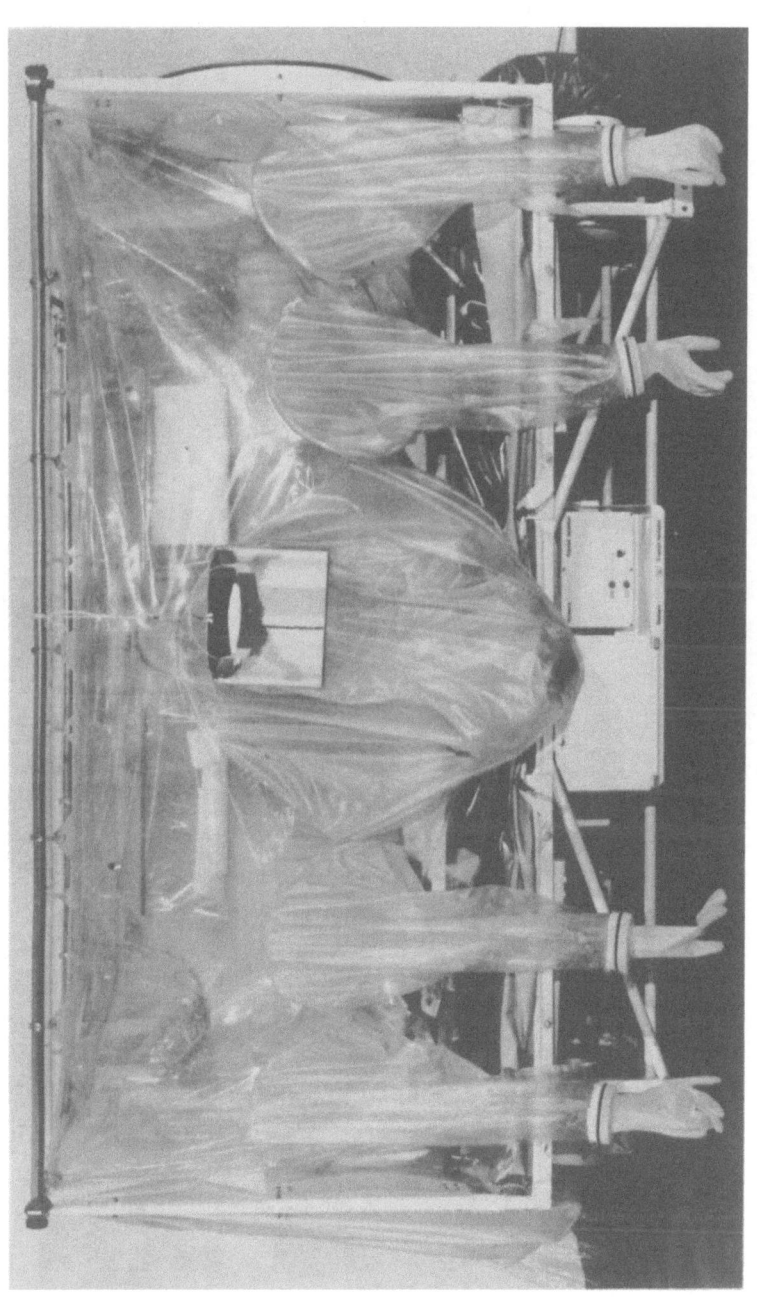

Figure 7

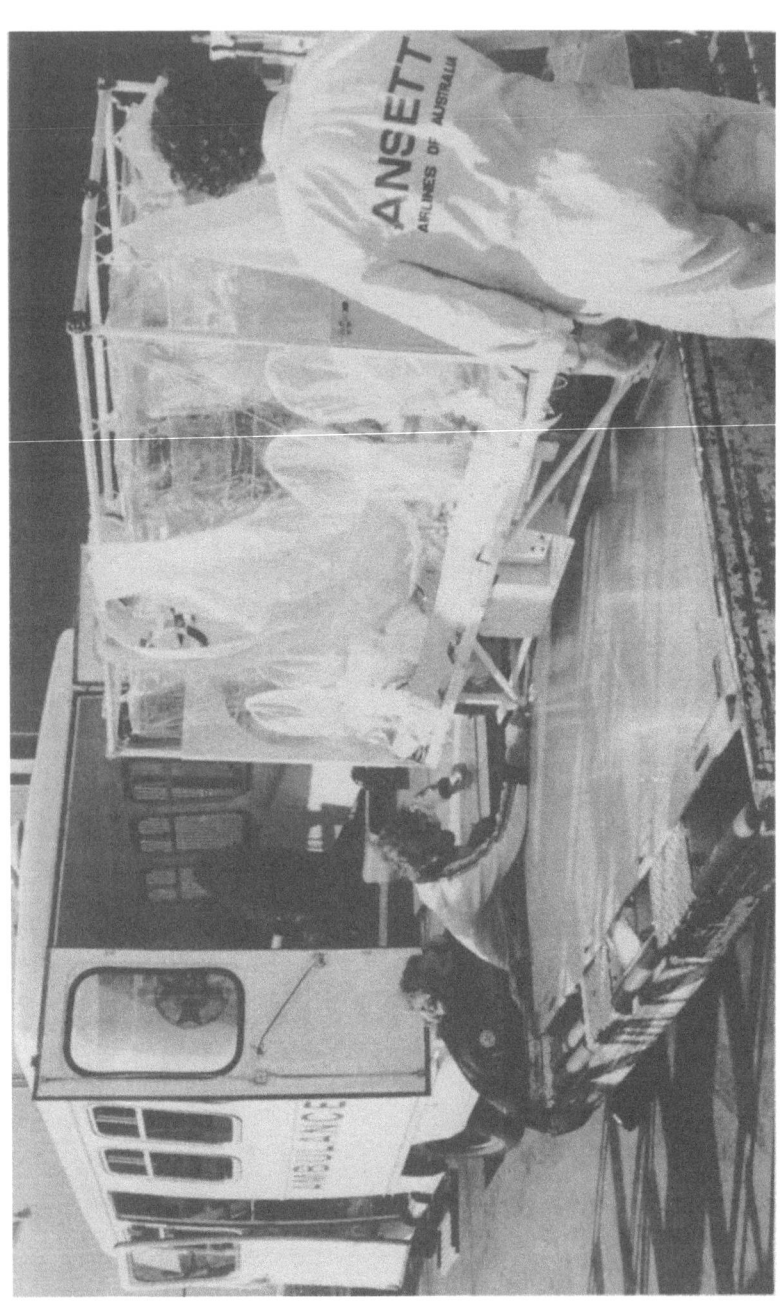

Figure 8

To facilitate the safe movement of patients, the Vickers Medical Company, in collaboration with Canadian Armed Forces, National Defence Medical Centre, has developed two types of transport isolator: the Air Transit Isolator (ATI) (see Figure 7) for distance transit by aircraft, and a smaller Stretcher Transit Isolator (STI) (see Figure 8) for short journeys by ambulance. A prototype of the ATI, supplied by the Canadian Government, was used to evacuate a sick US Peace Corps worker from Zaire to Johannesburg during the Ebola fever epidemic of 1976, and a more developed version[131] has now been adopted in both Canada and Australia. Australia holds 12 ATIs at various key ports of entry.

Long-distance transportation of a seriously ill patient, especially one suffering from vomiting and diarrhoea, could not be undertaken without difficulty and even serious risk to the patient. The movement of patients within the country is likely to be restricted to short distances in the early stages of the disease when the patient is still clinically robust. This restriction carries the implication that, either by reason of distance or of the clinical condition of the patient, a community hospital may be committed to the management of a VHF patient for the full duration of his illness. This suggests that it might be desirable to locate reserve bed-isolators at strategic points across the country so that they would be easily and rapidly available to community hospitals in all areas.

Laboratory. All specimens taken from the patient for laboratory examination must be regarded as being highly infective. Blood is likely to contain high concentrations of virus so any materials, such as faeces, which may be contaminated with blood are likely to be dangerous. Viruria is frequent and body fluids and exudates are infective.

Handling such specimens in a normal diagnostic laboratory is a dangerous procedure, so specimens taken for laboratory examination should be kept to the minimum required for establishing a diagnosis and for patient management.

The following specimens *must* be taken:

1. Thick and thin blood films for exclusion of malaria;
2. blood for haematology for determination of WBC and differential count;

3. blood cultures for bacteriology for exclusion of typhoid fever and other causes of septicaemia;
4. stool for bacterial culture for exclusion of *typhoid salmonellosis*;
5. urine for bacterial culture for exclusion of pyelitis;
6. throat swabs for bacterial culture for exclusion of *streptococceal pharyngitis* and *candidiasis*;
7. blood in EDTA containers for virus isolation;
8. throat swabs or washings for virus isolation.

Specimens 1 through 6 should be examined locally by the hospital diagnostic laboratory. Specimens 7 and 8 must be sent to a designated high-security laboratory for viral studies.

In addition to these specimens, it is likely that biochemical and additional haematological data are desirable for diagnosis or for monitoring clinical progress. Special arrangements may have to be made for handling such specimens and these should be anticipated *before* the need arises.

The problems of safety in diagnostic laboratories arise largely because technologists in biochemistry, haematology and general pathology sections do not think in terms of the possible microbial content of specimens which they handle and tend to treat them as inert reagents. It is not natural for them to take the elementary precautions which are second nature to microbiologists, and in any hospital diagnostic laboratory close examination of technical procedures will reveal gross discrepancies in terms of safe handling of parallel specimens from a single patient being examined by different sections. An obvious example would be blood from a patient with PUO who eventually proved to have a *Salmonella typhi* bacteriaemia. The same blood would be treated with markedly different degrees of respect in the various sections of the laboratory, and the urine from the same patient would probably be examined in a purely routine manner in urinalysis.

This situation has improved to some extent since laboratory infections with Hepatitis B have underlined the danger of laboratory specimens but even now there are very few hospital diagnostic laboratories in which all routine blood work is carried out in safety cabinets with the technician's hands protected by gloves, or even under exhaust-ventilated bench hoods.

The mechanical and automated equipment now universally used in biochemistry and haematology was designed by engineers with no consideration of infective hazard. A good example is the slide spinner designed to produce an even blood film for haematological examination. The slide is situated horizontally upon a flat rotor and a small pool of blood placed at its centre. The lid is then closed and the slide spun at high speed flinging the blood off by centrifugal force to leave a monocellular film adhering to the slide. The instrument operates in a manner closely resembling the spinning-disc apparatus designed at Porton in 1960 to produce monodispersed aerosols for biological warfare studies. A further danger lies in the way the resulting blood film extends to the very edges of the slide so that the slide cannot be handled without contaminating the fingers. With VHF blood, such contamination would be excessively dangerous. This kind of instrumentation may be safely used only with full knowledge of each and every hazard involved.

To add to the danger, it is very likely that the first case admitted to a general hospital will not be suspected until the second week when failure to respond to therapy and the emergence of more characteristic signs and symptoms will provoke clinical reassessment. By that time, many laboratory investigations will have been completed without special precautions.

It would seem wise for hospitals and public health laboratories which carry out diagnostic examinations to examine the microbiological safety of their procedures to ensure that the diagnosis of the index case is not made as a result of the death of a pathologist or technician. The task is not made easier by the fact that today there are no generally accepted safety standards for diagnostic laboratories.

The standards which have recently been drawn up by medical research councils and equivalent bodies on both sides of the Atlantic have been designed for research laboratories working with specified materials and infectious agents. They are, moreover, primarily concerned with containment – that is, preventing the escape of the organism from the laboratory – rather than the safety of the research personnel. They cannot be indiscriminately applied to diagnostic laboratories which do not know the nature of the agent they are working with until after the event. Logically, such laboratories should always have their staff work under the highest category of containment using effective biological safety-cabinets and wearing full protective clothing. Since this is impossible, it is inevitable that in the laboratory area an element of risk must be accepted. This should, however, be reduced to a minimum by detailed examination of instrumentation and procedures to identify and correct or circumvent specific risk factors, by using simple exhaust-ventilated bench hoods and having staff use basic personal protection by gown and gloves where appropriate. Such measures should be reinforced by a code of general hygienic behaviour and by changing overalls, which should be colour-coded, when leaving the laboratory area for visits to the hospital floors or the cafeteria.

13

Final Discussion

The study which this book is derived from was commissioned as a research project by the Ministry of Health of Ontario and supported by the Canadian Federal Health authorities of Health and Welfare Canada to help in establishing an appropriate level of response to the threat of importation of dangerous exotic communicable diseases. The stimulus was, of course, the threat from Lassa fever, reinforced by the Ebola fever epidemic of 1976, but the federal working party responsible for establishing a Canadian Contingency Plan also considered the possible threat from other communicable diseases which might conceivably cause uncontrollable epidemics.

From the evidence which has been presented, it may be concluded that, with the exception of yellow fever in tropical and sub-tropical zones, none of the diseases studied present a significant epidemic threat to developed communities. They do, however, present a very real threat to health care personnel. Consequently, it may be confidently expected that simple public health precautions would prevent epidemic spread, but that very positive action would be required to prevent nosocomial infections, especially infections among nursing and medical staff. The extent of such action must be determined on the basis of a number of factors based upon social and political acceptability.

Potentially threatening diseases may be divided into five categories.

1. Known diseases sufficiently studied to permit a reasonable assessment of the present threat.
2. Known diseases where foreseeable changes could bring about a dramatic escalation of threat.

3. Diseases which might develop an epidemic threat with longer term evolutionary changes.
4. New diseases yet to be encountered.
5. Diseases which have achieved epidemiological prominence and attracted global interest to the extent that they have become politically sensitive issues.

These categories are by no means mutually exclusive.

Into the first category fall the diseases considered in detail in Section Two. Lassa and Ebola fevers also fall into the second category. Their low person-to-person transmissibility is directly dependent upon their low transmissibility by the respiratory route, a characteristic which could be changed as a result of a minor alteration in tropism. This potential has probably already been seen in the Jos hospital outbreak of Lassa fever in 1970 (see p. 71).

The third category represents the more speculative possibilities of longer term evolutionary changes such as those exhibited by Rift Valley fever and dengue haemorrhagic fever, and the possible re-emergence of smallpox from such viruses as monkey pox and white-pox maintained in unknown animal reservoirs.

The fourth category is that of unknown disease, probably of viral aetiology and certainly of zoonotic origin still to be uncovered by human invasion of wilderness areas. No reasonable speculation is possible regarding such diseases.

The fifth category is the most potent in determining the nature and degree of public health response. While the annual death-toll from road accidents is accepted by society with concern, and that from influenza, running into thousands each year, with minor interest, the occurrence of a single death from Lassa fever transmitted in a developed community would be enough to initiate a near-panic from fear of the unknown and to have far-reaching political repercussions. It is this social and political fear which will trigger action if a true emergency occurs.

Appendix

The differential diagnosis of Lassa and Marburg-Ebola fevers in travellers from Africa with pyrexia of unknown origin.

A wide range of tropical infections causing fever, malaise and prostration are endemic in the regions of Africa where Lassa and Marburg-Ebola fevers occur. For instance, at the time of the Zaire outbreak of Ebola fever, the following infectious diseases were found to be endemic in the area: amoebiasis; dysentery; filariasis; malaria; measles; pneumonia and tuberculosis. A variety of known and probably unknown arbovirus infections such as yellow fever, dengue, Congo-Crimean fever, Rift Valley fever and Chikungunya fever must also be considered.

In practice, the range of likely disease in all but long-time residents in Africa is more restricted and British experience suggests that malaria and respiratory infections are by far the most common causes of PUO in travellers.

Clinical presentation, in cases other than those caused by pure anxiety, is likely to involve a series of non-specific 'influenza-like' symptoms; the most constant signs are fever, malaise, headache and muscle pains. Signs of respiratory tract involvement such as pharyngitis and pneumonitis with cough may be present early or may develop. Signs of gastro-intestinal involvement such as vomiting, diarrhoea and abdominal pain and tenderness may also be present. Differential diagnosis should, therefore, cover the following possibilities:

Malaria
Bacterial pharyngitis and pneumonia
Bacterial or enteroviral gastro-enteritis

Typhoid fever
Urinary tract infection
Influenza
Bacteriaemia or septicaemia due to a variety of underlying
   causes.

This list suggests that laboratory investigation should cover
the specimens and examinations given in Table 13.

TABLE 13   Suggested laboratory investigation

Specimen	Investigation	Disease
Throat swab	Culture	Bacterial pharyngitis
Blood	Thick and thin films for microscopy	Malaria Filariasis

	Culture (bacterial)	Typhoid fever
		Bacteriaemia and
		   septicaemia from
		   other causes

	Culture (viral)	Lassa and Ebola fevers

	White cell count and differential	Bacterial infection
		   (Leucotytosis)
		Lassa fever
		   (Leucopaenia)

	Serology (HB$_s$Ag)	Hepatitis B
Stool	Microscopy	Parasitic infestation
	Culture	Typhoid fever Salmonellosis Shigellosis Campylobacter enteritis
Urine	Urinalysis and culture	Urinary tract infection

Other serological investigations for typhoid, influenza, infectious mononucleosis or other possible infections may also be
included but if viral haemorrhagic fever is a real possibility,
such investigations and also biochemical and haematological

tests should be avoided as far as possible so as to reduce the risk to attendant staff and laboratory personnel.

The most critical immediate tests are the examination of thick and thin blood films for malaria since delay in the treatment of *P. falciparum* malaria may be fatal. It must be remembered, though, that since malaria is so common, the presence of malarial infection does not in itself exclude other infectious disease including VHF. In such cases, precautions should not be relaxed until the clinical condition shows an adequate response to anti-malarial therapy.

Finally, it must be remembered that all laboratory specimens are potentially hazardous and must be handled only by skilled staff who are fully aware of the dangers and who work under the safest conditions which can be locally devised. All laboratory investigations, both for diagnosis and for clinical management, should be kept to a minimum.[165, 181, 185]

Bibliography

Smallpox

1. F. Fenner. In 'Medical Virology', Academic Press Inc., N.Y. and London, second ed. (1976), 102–106.
2. H. M. Gelfand and J. Posch. The recent outbreak of smallpox in Meschede, West Germany. *Am. J. Epidemiol.*, **93** (1971), 234–237.
3. D. A. Henderson. The eradication of smallpox. *Scientific American* **235** (1976), 25–33.
4. D. A. Henderson. The saga of smallpox eradication. *Can. J. Pub. Hlth.*, **70** (1979), 21–28.
5. US Public Health Service. Morbidity and Mortality Weekly Reps. Compiled from WHO Weekly Epidemiological Records, **45**, 23 (20 June 1970) 249–256.
6. J. C. N. Westwood. Smallpox in Bradford. *Proc. Roy. Soc. Med.*, **56** (1962), 346–347.
7. J. C. N. Westwood and S. A. Sattar. The minimal infective dose, in *Viruses in Water*. American Public Health Association, G. Berg *et al.* eds. (1976), pp. 61–69.
8. World Health Organization. *Monkey-pox and white poxviruses in West and Central Africa* (1976), WHO/SE/76–78.
9. World Health Organization. *Report of informal consultation on monkey pox, whitepox and related poxviruses.* S.M.E. **78** (1978), 20.

Yellow fever

10. J. B. Blake. Yellow fever in eighteenth century America. *Bull. N.Y. Acad. Med.*, **44** (1968), 673–686.
11. D. E. Carey *et al.* Epidemiological aspects of the 1969 yellow fever epidemic in Nigeria. *Bull. WHO*, **46** (1972), 645–651.
12. W. G. Downs. The story of yellow fever since Walter Reed. *Bull. N.Y. Acad. Med.*, **44** (1968), 721–727.

13. J. Duffy. Yellow fever in the continental United States during the nineteenth century. *Bull. N.Y. Acad. Med.*, **44** (1968), 687–701.

14. A. J. Haddow *et al.* Yellow fever in Central Uganda. *Trans. Roy. Soc. Trop. Med. Hyg.*, **59** (1965), No. 4.
     Part I Haddow *et al.* Historical introduction, 436–440.
     Part II J. A. Tulloch and K. M. Patel. Report of a fatal case, 441–443.
     Part III M. C. Williams *et al.* Virus isolation from man and laboratory studies, 444–448.
     Part IV D. I. H. Simpson *et al.*, Investigations on blood-sucking diptera and monkeys, 449–458.

15. A. J. Haddow and J. M. Ellice. Studies on bush-babies (Galago species) with special reference to the epidemiology of yellow fever. *Trans. Roy. Soc. Trop. Med. Hyg.*, **58** (1964) 521–538.

16. B. E. Henderson *et al.* Modification of clinical response (to yellow fever) in vervet monkeys by immunization with Zika virus. *Amer. J. Epidemiol.*, **91** (1970), 87–98.

17. H. H. Scott. A history of tropical medicine: based on the Fitzpatrick lectures delivered before the Royal College of Physicians of London, 1937–8. Williams & Wilkins Co. (1939), Baltimore.

18. C. Série *et al.* Epidemic of yellow fever in Ethiopia 1960–62 (Abstract). *Trop. Dis. Bull.*, **62** (1965), 96.

19. F. L. Soper. *Aedes aegypti* and yellow fever. *Bull. WHO.*, **36** (1967), 521–527.

20. L. Spence *et al.* Yellow fever in two patients with pre-existing group B antibodies. *W. Ind. Med. J.*, **10** (1961), 54–58.

21. G. K. Strode *et al. Yellow Fever.* G. K. Strode (ed.), McGraw-Hill, 1951, N.Y.

22. World Health Organization.
     (a) Yellow fever in Ethiopia. *WHO Chronicle*, **18** (1964), 390–2
     (b) Expert Committe on Yellow Fever. 3rd Report, WHO Technical Report Series, **479** (1971), 1–56
     (c) 'Yellow Fever'. *WHO Chronicle*, **26** (1972), 60–65.

Dengue haemorrhagic fever

23. S. B. Halstead. Dengue and haemorrhagic fevers in Southeast Asia. *Yale J. Biol. Med.*, **37** (1965), 434–454.

24. W. McD. Hammon *et al.* Viruses associated with epidemic haemorrhagic fevers of the Philippines and Thailand. *Science*, **131** (1960), 1102–1103.

Rift Valley fever

25. K. S. E. Abdel-Wahab *et al.* Rift Valley fever virus infections in Egypt: Pathological and virological findings in man. *Trans. R. Soc. Trop. Med. Hyg.*, **72** (1979), 392–396.

26. R. Daubney *et al.* Enzootic hepatitis or Rift Valley fever. An undescribed virus disease of sheep, cattle and man from East Africa. *J. Path Bact.*, **34** (1931), 545–579.
27. F. G. Davies. Observations on the epidemiology of Rift Valley fever in Kenya. *J. Hyg. (Camb.)*, **75** (1975), 219–230.
28. F. G. Davies *et al.* The pathogenicity of RVF virus for the baboon. *Trans. R. Soc. Trop. Med. Hyg.*, **66** (1972), 363–365.
29. J. Gear *et al.* Rift Valley fever in South Africa. *S. Africa Med. J.*, **29** (1955), 514–518.
30. B. K. Johnson *et al.* Rift Valley fever in Egypt. *Lancet II* (1978), 745.
31. D. J. J. Van Delden *et al.* Rift Valley fever affecting humans in S. Africa. *S. Afr. Med. J.*, **51** (1977), 867–871.
32. World Health Organization. 1977–78. Rift Valley Fever in Egypt. Weekly Epidemiol. Record., 1977, §50:401; 1978, §1:7–8; 1978, §27:197–198.

Other haemorrhagic fevers

33. J. Casals *et al.* A review of Soviet viral haemorrhagic fevers (1969). *J. Infect. Dis.*, **122** (1970), 437–453.
34. J. Casals *et al.* A current appraisal of haemorrhagic fevers in the USSR. *Am. J. Trop. Med. Hyg.*, **15** (1966), 751–764.
35. K. M. Johnson *et al.* Haemorrhagic fevers of Southeast Asia and South America: A comparative appraisal. *Prog. Med. Virol.*, **9** (1967), 105–158.
36. M. D. Kastello *et al.* A rhesus monkey model for the study of Bolivian fever. *J. Infect Dis.*, **133** (1976), 57–62.
37. K. H. Kim *et al.* Recent epidemiological features on Korean haemorrhagic fever in the Republic of Korea. *Int. J. Zoonoses*, **4** (1977), 87–102.
38. H. P. Lambert. Personal discussion.
39. R. B. MacKenzie *et al.* Epidemic haemorrhagic fever in Bolivia, I. A preliminary report of the epidemiologic and clinical findings in a new epidemic area in South America. *Am. J. Trop. Med. Hyg.*, **13** (1964), 620–625.
40. J. I. Maiztegui. Clinical and epidemiological patterns of Argentine haemorrhagic fever. *Bull. WHO*, **52** (1975), 567–575.
41. R. Mercado. Rodent control programmes in areas affected by Bolivian haemorrhagic fever. *Bull. WHO*, **52** (1975), 691–696.
42. D. I. H. Simpson. Viral haemorrhagic fevers of man. *Bull. WHO*, **56** (1978), 819–832.
43. P. A. Webb *et al.* Infection of wild and laboratory animals with Machupo and Latino viruses. *Bull. WHO*, **52** (1975), 493–499.
44. M. C. Weinenbacher. Experimental biology and pathogenesis of Junin virus infection in animals and man. *Bull. WHO*, **52** (1975), 507–515.

Lassa fever

45. Arenaviruses in perspective (editorial). *Br. Med. J.*, 1 (1978), 529–530.
46. R. B. Arnold and G. W. Gary. A neutralization test survey for Lassa Nigeria. *Trans. R. Soc. Trop. Med. Hyg.*, 71 (1977), 152–154.
47. E. W. Best. The Lassa fever episode, Metro Toronto, August 1976. *Can J. Pub. Hlth.*, 67 (1976), 361–366, 369–374.
48. A. Bloch. A serological survey of Lassa fever in Liberia. *Bull. WHO*, 56 (1978), 811–813.
49. G. S. Bowen *et al.* Lassa fever in Onitsha, East Central State, Nigeria, 1974. *Bull. WHO*, 52 (1975), 599–604.
49a. Paul Brès. Personal communication.
50. S. M. Buckley. Lassa fever, a new virus disease of man from West Africa. III. Isolation and characterization of the virus. *Am. J. Trop. Med. Hyg.*, 19 (1970), 680–681.
51. D. E. Carey. Lassa fever: Epidemiological aspects of the 1970 epidemic, Jos, Nigeria. *Trans. Roy. Soc. Trop. Med. Hyg.*, 66 (1972), 402–408.
52. J. Casals. Lassa fever. *Progr. Med. Virol.*, 18 (1974), 111–126.
53. J. Casals *et al.* Antigenic properties of the arenaviruses. *Bull. WHO*, 52 (1975), 421–428.
54. A. J. Clayton. Lassa immune serum. *Bull. WHO*, 55 (1977), 435–439.
55. G. M. Edington and H. A. White. The pathology of Lassa fever. *Trans. Roy. Soc. Trop. Med. Hyg.*, 66 (1972), 381–389.
56. T. C. Eickhoff. Containing Andromeda (editorial). *N. Eng. J. Med.*, 297 (1977), 835–836.
57. A. Fabiyi. Lassa fever (arenaviruses) as a public health problem. *Bull. Pan. Am. Hlth. Organ.*, 10 (1976), 335–337.
58. J. D. Frame *et al.* Lassa fever, a new virus disease of man from West Africa. Clinical description and pathological features. *Am. J. Trop. Med. Hyg.*, 19 (1970), 670–676.
59. J. D. Frame *et al.* Lassa virus antibodies in hospital personnel in Western Liberia. *Trans. Roy. Soc. Trop. Med. Hyg.*, 73 (1979), 219–224.
60. D. W. Fraser *et al.* Lassa fever in the Eastern Province of Sierra Leone 1970–72. Epidemiological studies. *Am. J. Trop. Med. Hyg.*, 23 (1974), 1131.
61. J. G. Fuller. *Fever! The hunt for a new killer virus.* London (1974), Hart-Davis, MacGibbon.
62. H. M. Gilles and J. C. Kent. Lassa fever: Retrospective diagnosis of two patients seen in Great Britain in 1971. *Br. Med. J.*, 2 (1976), 1173.
63. M. B. Gregg. Recent outbreaks of lymphocytic choriomeningitis in the United States of America. *Bull. WHO*, 52 (1975), 549–554.

64. M. H. Hambling *et al.* Decreasing any viral infectivity in blood-smears for malarial parasite examination (letter). *Lancet,* 1 (1978), 222.
65. B. E. Henderson *et al.* Lassa fever: virological and serological studies. *Trans. Roy. Soc. Trop. Med. Hyg.,* 66 (1972), 409–416.
66. International Symposium on Arenaviral Infections of Public Health Importance. *Bull. WHO,* 52 (1975), 381–765.
67. M. Isaacson. The ecology of *Praomys. (Mastomys.) natalensis* in Southern Africa. *Bull. WHO,* 52 (1975), 629–636.
68. K. M. Johnson. Status of arenavirus vaccines and their application. *Bull. WHO,* 52 (1975), 729–736.
69. K. M. Johnson. The arenaviruses: Some priorities for future research. *Bull. WHO,* 52 (1975), 761–764.
70. E. Keane and H. M. Gilles. Lassa fever in Panguma Hospital, Sierra Leone, 1973–76. *Br. Med. J.,* 1 (1977), 1399–1402.
71. E. Leifer. Lassa fever, a new virus disease of man from West Africa. II. Report of a laboratory-acquired infection treated with plasma from a person recently recovered from the disease. *Am. J. Trop. Med. Hyg.,* 19 (1970), 677–679.
72. J. B. McCormick and K. M. Johnson. Lassa fever: historical review and contemporary investigation. In: *Ebola Virus Haemorrhagic Fever.* S. R. Pattyn, (ed.), (1978), Elsevier, Amsterdam–New York, 279–286.
73. J. I. Maiztequi. Clinical and epidemiological patterns of Argentinian haemorrhagic fever. *Bull. WHO,* 52 (1975), 567–576.
74. P. E. Mertens. Clinical presentation of Lassa fever cases during the hospital epidemic at Zorzor, Liberia, March–April 1972. *Am. J. Trop. Med. Hyg.,* 22 (1973), 780–784.
75. T. P. Monath. A hospital epidemic of Lassa fever in Zorzor, Liberia, March–April 1972. *Am. J. Trop. Med. Hyg.,* 22 (1973), 773–779.
76. T. P. Monath *et al.* Lassa fever in the Eastern Province of Sierra Leone, 1970–72. II. Clinical observations and virological studies on selected hospital cases. *Am. J. Trop. Med. Hyg.,* 23 (1974), 1140–1149.
77. T. P. Monath. Lassa fever and Marburg virus disease. *WHO Chron.,* 28 (1974), 212–219.
78. T. P. Monath and J. Casals. Diagnosis of Lassa fever and the isolation and management of patients. *Bull. WHO,* 52 (1975), 707–716.
79. T. P. Monath. Lassa fever: review of epidemiology and epizootiology. *Bull. WHO* 52 (1975), 577–592.
80. F. A. Murphy. Arenavirus taxonomy: A review. *Bull. WHO,* 52 (1975), 389–391.
81. F. A. Murphy and S. G. Whitfield. Morphology and morphogenesis of arenaviruses. *Bull. WHO,* 52 (1975), 409–419.
82. J. Owen. Lassa fever surveillance: The need for better communication. *Can. J. Pub. Hlth.,* 68 (1977), 101–105.

83. C. J. Pfau. Biochemical and biophysical properties of the arenaviruses. *Progr. Med. Virol.*, **18** (1974), 64–80.
84. Report CDC, Atlanta, *M.M.W.R.*, **21** (1972), 237–238.
85. Report, Memorandum on Lassa fever. (1976), London, HMSO.
86. W. P. Rowe. Arenaviruses: Proposed name for a newly defined virus group. *J. Virol.*, **5** (1970), 651–652.
87. S. K. Seah. Lassa, Marburg and Ebola: Newly described African fevers (editorial). *Can. Med. Assoc. J.*, **118** (1978), 347–348, 350.
88. E. A. Smith. A review of Lassa fever outbreaks in Nigeria. *Nigerian Med. J.*, **4** (1974), 216.
89. R. W. Speir. Lassa fever, a new virus disease of man from West Africa. IV. Electron microscopy of vero cell cultures infected with Lassa virus. *Am. J. Trop. Med. Hyg.*, **19** (1970), 692–696.
90. E. L. Stephen and P. B. Jahrling. Experimental Lassa fever virus infection successfully treated with Ribavirin. *Lancet* 1 (1979), 268–269.
91. J. M. Troup. An outbreak of Lassa fever on the Jos Plateau, Nigeria, in Jan–Feb 1970. A preliminary report. *Am. J. Trop. Med. Hyg.*, **19** (1970), 695–696.
92. E. E. Vella. Lassa fever. *Hospital Update*, **2** (1976), 31.
93. D. H. Walker *et al.* Comparative pathology of Lassa virus infection in monkeys, guinea-pigs and *Mastomys natalensis*. *Bull. WHO*, **52** (1975), 523–545.
94. H. A. White. Lassa fever: A study of 23 hospital cases. *Trans. Roy. Soc. Trop. Med. Hyg.*, **66** (1972), 390–398.
95. W. C. Winn and D. H. Walker. The pathology of human Lassa fever. *Bull. WHO*, **52** (1975), 535–545.
96. A. W. Woodruff *et al.* Lassa fever in Britain: An imported case. *Br. Med. J.*, **3** (1973), 616–617.
97. H. Wulff *et al.* Recent isolation of Lassa virus from Nigerian rodents. *Bull. WHO*, **52** (1975), 609–614.
98. H. Wulff *et al.* Isolation of an arenavirus closely related to Lassa virus from *Mastomys natalensis* in South-East Africa. *Bull. WHO*, **55** (1977), 441–444.
99. A. J. Zuckerman. Lassa fever and public health. *Nature* (London), **251** (1974), 101–102.
100. R. M. Zweighaft *et al.* Lassa fever: Response to an imported case. *N. Engl. J. Med.*, **297** (1977), 803–807.

Ebola-Marburg fever

101. J. D. Almeida *et al.* Morphology and morphogenesis of the Marburg agent. In *Marburg Virus Disease*, G. A. Martini and R. Siegert (eds.). (1971), Springer-Verlag, Berlin and New York, 84–97.

102. E. T. W. Bowen. 1978 characterization and epidemiology of viruses belonging to the African haemorrhagic fever group with particular reference to Marburg type viruses. Ph.D. thesis, Special Pathogens Division, M.R.E. Porton, Salisbury, Wilts., England.

103. E. T. W. Bowen *et al.* Vervet monkey disease: Studies on some physical and chemical properties of the causative agent. *Brit. J. Exp. Path.*, **50** (1969), 400–407.

104. E. T. W. Bowen *et al.* Viral haemorrhagic fever in Southern Sudan and Northern Zaire. Preliminary studies on the aetiological agent. *Lancet* **1** (1977), 571–573.

105. E. T. W. Bowen *et al.* Ebola haemorrhagic fever: Experimental infection of monkeys. *Trans. Roy. Soc. Trop. Med. Hyg.*, **72** (1978), 188–191.

106. J. Casals. Absence of serological relationship between Marburg virus and some arboviruses. In *Marburg Virus Disease*, G. A. Martini and R. Siegert (eds.). (1971), Springer-Verlag, Berlin and New York, 98.

107. L. Clausen *et al.* Isolation and handling of patients with dangerous infectious disease. *S. Afr. Med. J.*, **53** (1978), 238–242.

108. J. L. Conrad *et al.* Epidemiological investigation of Marburg virus disease, Southern Africa, 1975. *Am. J. Trop. Med. Hyg.*, **27** (1978), 1210–15.

109. D. S. Ellis *et al.* Ebola virus: A comparison, at ultrastructural level, of the behaviour of the Sudan and Zaire strains in monkeys. *Br. J. Exp. Path.*, **59** (1978), 584–593.

110. D. S. Ellis *et al.* Ultrastructure of Ebola virus particles in human liver. *J. Clin. Pathol.*, **31** (1978), 201–208.

111. R. T. Emond *et al.* A case of Ebola virus infection. *Br. Med. J.*, **2** (1977), 541–544.

112. J. S. S. Gear *et al.* Outbreak of Marburg virus disease in Johannesburg. *Br. Med. J.*, **4** (1975), 489–493.

113. J. H. Gear. Haemorrhagic fevers of Africa: An account of two recent outbreaks. *J. S. Afr. Vet. Assoc.*, **48** (1977), 5–8.

114. E. D. Gomperts *et al.* Handling of highly infectious material in a clinical pathology laboratory and in a viral diagnostic unit. *S. Afr. Med. J.*, **53** (1978), 243–248.

115. R. Haas and G. Maass. Experimental infection of monkeys with the Marburg virus. In *Marburg Virus Disease*, G. A. Martini and R. Siegert (eds.). (1971), Springer-Verlag, Berlin and New York, 136–143.

116. B. E. Henderson *et al.* Epidemiological studies in Uganda relating to the 'Marburg' agent. In *Marburg Virus Disease*, G. A. Martini and R. Siegert (eds.). (1971), Springer-Verlag, Berlin and New York, 166–176.

117. W. Hennessen. Epidemiology of 'Marburg Virus' disease. In *Marburg Virus Disease*, G. A. Martini and R. Siegert (eds.). (1971), Springer-Verlag, Berlin and New York, 161–165.

118. An isolated case of Marburg. *Nurs. Times*, **73** (1977), 262–263.
119. K. M. Johnson *et al.* Isolation and partial characterization of a new virus causing acute haemorrhagic fever in Zaire. *Lancet* **1** (1977), 569–571.
120. S. S. Kalter. A serological survey of primate sera for antibody to the Marburg virus. In *Marburg Virus Disease*, G. A. Martini and R. Siegert (eds.) (1971). Springer-Verlag, Berlin and New York, 177–187.
121. C. Kunz *et al.* Propagation of the Marburg Virus in *Aedes aegypti. Zbl. Bakt. I. Orig.*, **208** (1968), 344–347.
122. H. Malherbe and M. Strickland-Cholmley. Studies on the Marburg virus. In *Marburg Virus Disease*, G. A. Martini and R. Siegert (eds.) (1971). Springer-Verlag, Berlin and New York, 188–194.
123. G. A. Martini and R. Siegert (eds.). *Marburg Virus Disease* (1971). Springer-Verlag, Berlin and New York.
124. G. A. Martini. Marburg agent disease: In man. *Trans. Roy. Soc. Trop. Med. Hyg.*, **63** (1969) 295.
125. G. A. Martini. Marburg Virus Disease. Clinical syndrome. In *Marburg Virus Disease*, G. A. Martini and R. Siegert (eds.) (1971). Springer-Verlag, Berlin and New York, 1–9.
126. G. A. Martini *et al.* Spermatogenic transmission of virus Marburg (1968). Wiener Klinische Wochenschrift.
127. S. Pattyn *et al.* Isolation of Marburg-like virus from a case of haemorrhagic fever in Zaire. *Lancet* **1** (1977), 573–574.
128. Report WHO. *Bull. WHO*, **56** (1978), 245–294.
      (a) P. Brès. Introductory note, 245.
      (b) Ebola haemorrhagic fever in Sudan, 1976, 247–270.
      (c) Ebola haemorrhagic fever in Zaire, 1976, 271–294.
129. R. Siegert and W. Schlenczka. Laboratory diagnosis and pathogenesis. In *Marburg Virus Disease*, G. A. Martini and R. Siegert (eds.) (1971). Springer-Verlag, Berlin and New York.
130. R. Siegert. Marburg virus. *Virology monographs 11* (1972). Springer-Verlag, Berlin and New York, p. 139.
131. D. I. H. Simpson *et al.*, Vervet monkey disease: Experimental infection of monkeys with the causative agent and antibody studies in wild-caught monkeys. *Lab. Anim.*, **2** (1968), 75–81.
132. D. I. H. Simpson. Marburg agent disease: In monkeys. *Trans. Roy. Soc. Trop. Med. Hyg.*, **63** (1969), 303–309.
133. D. I. H. Simpson. Marburg and Ebola virus infections: A guide to their diagnosis, management and control. Offset Publication No. 36, Geneva, (1977), WHO.
134. D. I. H. Simpson. Marburg virus: A review of laboratory studies. In *Infection and Immunosuppression in Subhuman Primates.* (1970). Munksgaard, Copenhagen.
135. C. E. G. Smith *et al.* Fatal human disease from vervet monkeys. *Lancet* ii (1967), 1119–1121.
136. C. E. G. Smith. Lessons from Marburg disease. *The Scientific Basis of Medicine Annual Reviews*, (1971), 58–80.

137. M. Strickland-Cholmley and H. Malherbe. Examination of South African primates for the presence of Marburg virus. In *Marburg Virus Disease*, G. A. Martini and R. Siegert (eds.) (1971). Springer-Verlag, Berlin and New York, 195–202.

138. K. Todarovitch *et al.* Clinical picture of two patients infected by the Marburg vervet virus. In *Marburg Virus Disease*, G. A. Martini and R. Siegert (eds.) (1971). Springer-Verlag, Berlin and New York, 19–23.

139. G. Van der Groen and S. R. Pattyn. Measurement of antibodies to Ebola virus in human sera from N.W. Zaire. *Ann. Soc. Belge, Med. Trop.*, **59** (1979), 87–92.

140. S. H. Williams. 44 contacts of Ebola virus infection – *Salisbury Public Health*, **93** (1979), 67–75.

Simian haemorrhagic fever

141. A. E. Palmer *et al.* Simian hemorrhagic fever. I. Clinical and epizootological aspects of an outbreak among quarantined monkeys. *Amer. J. Trop. Med. Hyg.*, **17** (1968), 404–412.

142. A. V. Shevtosva. Studies on the etiology of hemorrhagic fevers in monkeys. *Vop. Virusol.*, **12** (1967) 47–51.

143. N. M. Tauraso *et al.* Simian hemorrhagic fever. III. Isolation and characterization of a viral agent. *Amer. J. Trop. Med. Hyg.*, **17** (1968), 422–431.

Plague

144. G. Cravens and J. S. Marr. *The Black Death.* (1977), Weidenfeld and Nicolson Ltd., UK Futura Edition, (1978), Futura Publications Ltd., London.

145. H. A. Druett *et al.* Studies on respiratory infection. II. The influence of aerosol particle size on infection of the guinea-pig with *Pasteurella pestis. J. Hyg. (Camb.)*, **54** (1956), 37–48.

146. J. M. Mann. Plague pneumonia (letter). *New Eng. Med. J.*, (1979), 1276–77.

147. J. D. Marshall *et al.* Plague in Vietnam 1965–66. *Am. J. Epidemiol.*, **86** (1967), 603–616.

148. Plague. In *Principles of Bacteriology, Virology and Immunity.* (W.W.C. Topley & G. S. Wilson), 6th Ed., G. S. Wilson and S. A. Miles (eds.). Edward Arnold Ltd., London, 2120–2138.

149. J. D. Poland. Plague. In *Infectious Diseases*, P. D. Hoeprich (ed.) (1977). Harper & Row, N.Y.

150. A. Roberts. A history of plague in England. *Nursing Times*, (1979), 10 and 17 May.

151. J. F. D. Shrewsburg *A history of bubonic plague in the British Isles* (1970). Cambridge University Press: Cambridge, England.

152. WHO Expert Committee on Plague. *Technical Report Series No.* **447**, 1970.
153. P. Ziegler. *The Black Death*. Pelican Books, (1969). C. Nicholls & Co., Great Britain.

Legionnaires' disease

154. W. B. Baine. Legionnaires' disease: Epidemiology and clinical characteristics. In *Legionnaires, the disease, the bacterium and methodology* (1978). US Dept. of Hlth., Educ. and Welfare, Public Health Service, Center for Disease Control, Atlanta.
155. D. W. Fraser *et al.* Legionnaires' disease: Description of an epidemic. *New Engl. J. Med.*, **297** (197), 1189–1196.
156. T. H. Glick *et al.* Pontiac fever. An epidemic of unknown etiology in a health department. I. Clinical and epidemiological aspects. *Amer. J. Epidemiol.*, **107** (1978), 149–160.
157. Isolation of organisms resembling legionnaires' disease bacterium – Georgia (and editorial note). *M.M.W.R.*, **27** (1978), 415–416.
158. G. L. Jones and G. H. Herbert (eds.). *Legionnaires. The disease, the bacterium and methodology.* (1978), US Dept. of Hlth, Educ. and Welfare, Public Health Service, Center for Disease Control, Atlanta.
159. Legionnaires' Disease – Los Angeles, California. *M.M.W.R.*, **27** (1978), 394.
160. Legionnaires' Disease – United States. *M.M.W.R.*, **27** (1978), 439.
161. Legionnaires' Disease – Australia. *M.M.W.R.*, **27** (1979), 523.

General: Containment, Prophylaxis, Therapy, Reports and Editorial Comment

162. J. B. Brooksby. The control and eradication of exotic viruses affecting domestic animals. *Prog. Med. Virol.*, **25** (1979), 83–88.
163. A. J. Clayton. Lassa fever, Marburg and Ebola virus diseases and other exotic diseases. Is there a risk to Canada? *Can. Med. Assoc. J.*, **120** (1979), 146–152.
164. G. A. Eddy *et al.* Protection of monkeys against machupo virus by the passive administration of Bolivian haemorrhagic fever immunoglobulin (human origin). *Bull. WHO*, **52** (1975), 723–727.
165. R. T. Emond *et al.* Assessment of patients with suspected viral haemorrhagic fever. *Br. Med. J.*, 1 (1978), 966–967.
166. N. S. Galbraith *et al.* Public health aspects of viral haemorrhagic fevers in Britain. *Roy. Soc. Hlth. J.*, **98** (1978), 152–160.

167. J. H. Gear *et al*. A consideration of the diagnosis of dangerous infectious fevers in South Africa. *S. Afr. Med. J.*, **53** (1978), 235–237.

168. Health and Welfare Canada. 1978. Exotic Dangerous Communicable Diseases (Principles and Practices of Management), The Canadian Contingency Plan.

169. R. B. Hornick *et al*. Typhoid fever – pathogenesis and immunologic control. *New Eng. J. Med.*, **283** (1970), 686–691.

170. F. A. Murphy. Control and eradication of exotic viruses affecting man. *Prog. Med. Virol.*, **25** (1979), 69–82.

171. J. Owen. Lassa fever surveillance: The need for better communication. *Can. J. Pub. Hlth.*, **68** (1977), 101–105.

172. Report. The control of laboratory use in the United Kingdom of pathogens very dangerous to humans. (1976), DHSS and MAFF. London.

173. Report. On the state of the public health for the year 1975. London. (1976), HMSO, 41.

174. Report. On the state of the public health for the year 1976. London. (1977), HMSO, 52.

175. F. C. Robbins *et al*. Algorithms in the diagnosis and management of exotic diseases. XIX. Major tropical viral infections: Smallpox, yellow fever, and Lassa fever. *J. Infect. Dis.*, **135** (1977), 341–346.

176. P. C. Trexler *et al*. Negative-pressure plastic isolator for patients with dangerous infections. *Br. Med. J.*, **2** (1977), 559–561.

177. US Dept. Health, Education and Welfare. 1970. *Isolation techniques for use in hospitals. (Lassa fever ref.)*. Pub. Hlth. Service Publ. No. 2054, Washington, D.C.

178. Viral haemorrhagic fevers (editorial). *Publ. Hlth.*, **91** (1977), 3–5.

179. M. S. Wolfe. Containment of dangerous contagions (Letter). *N. Eng. J. Med.*, **297** (1977), 1355.

180. A. W. Woodruff. Handling patients with suspected Lassa fever entering Great Britain. *Bull. WHO*, **52** (1975), 717.

181. A. W. Woodruff *et al*. Viral infections in travellers from tropical Africa. *Br. Med. J.*, **1** (1978), 956–958.

182. World Health Organization. 1969. International Health Regulations. Geneva.

183. World Health Organization. Viral haemorrhagic fever. *Weekly Epidemiol. Record*, **52** (1977), 177 and 185.

Recent publications

184. Ebola Hemorrhagic Fever – Southern Sudan (International Notes). *M.M.W.R.*, **28**/No. 47 (1979), 557–559.

185. Recommendations for Initial Management of Suspected or Confirmed cases of Lassa Fever. *M.M.W.R.* (Supplement), **28**/No. 52 (1980), 3S–12S.